JOHN P. MARSDEN

Humanistic Design
of Assisted Living

THE JOHNS HOPKINS UNIVERSITY PRESS

BALTIMORE and LONDON

The Johns Hopkins University Press
2715 North Charles Street
Baltimore, Maryland 21218-4363
www.press.jhu.edu

Library of Congress Cataloging-in-Publication Data

Marsden, John P.
   Humanistic design of assisted living / John P. Marsden
      p. ; cm.
   Includes bibliographical references and index.
   ISBN 0-8018-8031-9 (pbk. : alk. paper)
   1. Nursing homes—design and construction. 2. Congregate housing—Design and
construction.
   [DNLM: 1. Assisted Living Facilities—Aged—United States. 2. Facility Design
and Construction—United States. WT 27 AA1 M264h 2005]   I. Title.
   RA998.5.M37 2005
   362.16—dc22   2004015974

A catalog record for this book is available from the British Library.

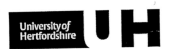

HUMANISTIC DESIGN OF ASSISTED LIVING

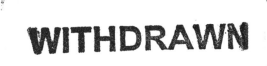

To Margaret, Will,

and my parents

CONTENTS

PREFACE

How Did This Book Evolve?

I have always been interested in older people. My curiosity was cultivated as a high school sophomore when my teacher Barbara Walsh required us students to contribute twenty hours of community service as part of a health education class at Saint John the Baptist Diocesan High School, on Long Island, New York. By the time I completed my senior year, I had not only satisfied the curriculum requirement at a local nursing home but also volunteered several hundred hours there. An undergraduate design studio at Carnegie Mellon University introduced me to the notion of integrating my interests in architecture and gerontology. As I worked on the assigned retirement housing project, however, I became increasingly frustrated with my lack of knowledge and the paucity of design resources available. I began to wonder how architects in their twenties, thirties, or even forties could effectively design environments for people in their eighties.

After several similar professional experiences at architecture firms, I returned to school to learn formally about housing for older adults. Dr. Dennis Doxtater introduced me to a research-oriented approach to design, and Linda Sanders supported my interest in environment and aging while I was at the University of Arizona. In a Ph.D. program in architecture at the University of Michigan, I became interested in strategies to obtain input from older adults about their design needs in assisted living and in ways to make research findings understandable and useful to designers. Dr. Rachel Kaplan showed me how the picture preference procedure could be used to obtain consumer input and address the research applicability gap. The studies of assisted living exterior entries and façades that serve as a foundation for this book were completed under her direction, with guidance from Dr. Kate Warner, as part of my dissertation work. As a generous mentor, Rachel also provided guidance with respect to environmental sampling and the interview procedure for the later studies that focused on interior spaces.

How Is the Book Organized?

This book consists of guidelines, based on several studies involving consumer input, for the humanistic design of assisted living. It includes eight chapters organized into three parts, along with an introduction and conclusion. The introduction discusses the studies that serve as a foundation for the guidelines. Part I provides background material. Chapter 1 discusses the evolution of assisted living and identifies reasons underlying its growth, such as exploding demographics among the oldest old, consumer demand for noninstitutional relocation alternatives, and fiscal concerns. The chapter also notes that assisted living is a confusing industry and reflects a wide range of providers, staffing, services, needs of residents, costs, and physical design attributes. Despite the diversity, the chapter attempts to identify common characteristics, services, and environmental features based on several national surveys conducted by industry organizations. Chapter 2 addresses resources available to guide the design of assisted living, distinguishing between resources that are weak and more subjective and those that are stronger in terms of validity and rigor. The dearth of research-based information that can be used to inform design decision making is attributed to the explosive growth of assisted living, diverse interpretations of research in architecture and interior design, and challenges associated with measuring the environment.

Part II is a discussion of humanistic design. Chapter 3 describes ways in which older adults and family members can provide input related to the design of assisted living through research, pointing out that consumer input is needed to support well-being and to compensate for differences in perception between designers and consumers. Currently, several obstacles hinder consumer input, including the lack of collaboration between consumers and designers, the insular education of designers and consumers, and the challenges of recruiting older people for research. The fourth chapter presents a conceptual framework that evolved from the studies and was used to develop the design guidelines. The framework comprises six overarching themes—familiar housing cues, protective enclosure, caring cues, human scale, usability, and naturalness—that help create a humane environment.

Part III consists of design guidelines based on results from several studies. The guidelines are grouped in chapters according to spaces and physical features that are familiar to those involved in the building development process. Chapter 5 focuses on exterior entries and building façades. Chapter 6 addresses interior entries, and chapters 7 and 8 focus on common shared spaces—living rooms and dining rooms, respectively. In each chapter, the design guidelines are organized in relation to the conceptual framework that evolved from the studies. Each construct of the framework can be considered a design goal. The highlighted statements under each design goal are more specific design recommendations. Design recommendations are described and supported by findings from the studies in tandem with photographs of existing buildings used during data collection. The photographs both demonstrate effective strategies for creating humane assisted living environments and point out features that were less successful from the consumer perspective. A photograph might be referred to throughout a chapter because each image can illustrate several features in the context of an entire façade or interior space.

The conclusion "puts it all together" by summarizing more than ninety design recommendations in tables that highlight relationships between the guidelines and the salient qualities comprising the humanistic design framework. There is a table for building exteriors and for each interior space. The tables provide a quick checklist for those involved in developing buildings for assisted living and illustrate how some of the design guidelines can work in tandem. The conclusion summarizes the similarities and differences between older adults and family members and stresses that some of the design recommendations may be applicable to other housing options for older adults, such as nursing homes and housing for independent living.

Who Helped along the Way?

In addition to my former instructors, several others assisted with the research that serves as a foundation for the book. Dr. Carol Warfield offered suggestions for my grant proposal to study assisted living interior spaces, which was subsequently funded by an Auburn University Competitive Research Grant and the Department of Consumer Affairs. I received help from many assisted living staff members and administrators with the recruitment of older participants and family members for the studies of both the exterior and interior spaces. Melanie Chastain and Madelen Raughton assisted with data collection for the interior studies. Most important are the older adults and family members who participated in the studies and made the research possible.

Many contributed to the development of this book. Wendy Harris, medical editor at the Johns Hopkins University Press, supported the book from the beginning and ensured its fruition. Dr. Maggie Calkins, always willing to help, offered advice about potential book publishers. Both Dr. John Scanzoni and Dr. Jo Hasell reviewed the initial book proposal and served as a sounding board for many ideas over an extended period. In addition to the anonymous reviewer, Dr. Jo Hasell evaluated the final manuscript. The College of Design, Construction, and Planning at the University of Florida provided some assistance for the writing of the book.

Family members offered help in other ways. My wife, Margaret, took a great interest in the book and reviewed early ideas. She has always supported my career choices with an optimistic and enthusiastic outlook. She also made it possible for me to work on my writing with minimal distractions. This was not always easy, especially when we learned that she was pregnant while I was writing chapter 2! My parents, Patrick and Helena, always encouraged me to further my education and strive to do my best. They have offered much financial and emotional support over the years and made it possible for me to pursue the career of my choice. My sister, Alexandra, and her husband, Jack, and sons, Kieran and Liam; my brother, Rob, and his wife, Kathy, and their children, Ryan and Matthew; my brother-in-law, Charlie, and his wife, Tamara; and family friend Martha all offered encouragement along the way.

HUMANISTIC DESIGN OF ASSISTED LIVING

INTRODUCTION

Many older Americans would like to age in their own homes. When this is not feasible, they must consider alternatives. One study has shown that moving in with family was not a desirable option for more than two-thirds of older Americans surveyed (American Association of Retired Persons [AARP], 1996). Relocating to a nursing home is not only an unwelcome choice but also a dreaded one. Assisted living, a relatively new industry, is being promoted as a favorable alternative to traditional long-term care, with emphasis on its resident-centered philosophy and noninstitutional environment. The research that serves as the basis for this book, however, indicates that older adults as well as family members do not always perceive the buildings used for assisted living as supportive or friendly.

This book is about the humanistic design of assisted living for consumers. Humanistic design entails consumer input. Older people in assisted living and family members who periodically visit should have a say about the environment. This is possible when consumers are asked about their needs and their perceptions of environments in the context of scientific research. Research-based information, translated into design guidelines that are easily applied by those without a research background, can be used to help architects and designers make more informed design decisions. Architects and designers are then more likely to create humane buildings that cultivate well-being and support consumers' abilities to function effectively.

This book is intended to serve as a guide for humanistic design to those involved in developing buildings for assisted living, including owners, operators, administrators, directors of marketing, architects, interior designers, gerontologists, policy makers, and researchers.

The Foundation for the Design Guidelines

The design guidelines in this book are derived from a series of small studies that elicited input from more than five hundred older adults and family members. The studies employed a method for obtaining consumer input called the picture preference procedure (Kaplan and Kaplan, 1989). Kaplan, Kaplan, and Wendt first used the picture preference procedure in 1972. Since then, many other researchers have used the procedure in several countries with diverse environmental settings and many different segments of the population. It has been used to a lesser degree with older adults.

In this procedure, participants view pictures of existing or simulated environments and indicate how much they like or dislike each picture using a five-point rating scale. The task is easy and even enjoyable for most people. Although photographs of environments are not the same as "being there," studies have demonstrated that responses to photographs of environments correlate highly with responses to actual environments (Feimer, 1984; Hershberger and Cass, 1988; Stamps, 1990). People can effectively draw inferences about visual features, spatial arrangements, and opportunities to function from two-dimensional pictures that represent three-dimensional environments. The popular use of pictures in travel brochures, for example, suggests that photographs provide a meaningful and understandable format for sharing information. Preference is also an effective way to measure what is important to people in the environment. Nasar (1999) reviewed thirty years of research findings that demonstrate strong commonalities in how people interpret built and natural environments. Shared needs and meanings have shown remarkable stability over time.

The strength of the method is derived from careful environmental sampling. It is important to include several instances of particular physical features to determine what aspects of the environment are preferred and how participants perceive the environment. The preference ratings can then be analyzed in multiple ways. Kaplan and Kaplan (1989) suggested that highly preferred scenes and strongly disliked scenes provide one type of information. Analysis techniques that extract clusters of items that group together based on correlations among ratings provide a second type of information about underlying perceptions. The photographs constituting a cluster or category reflect a common perceptual theme. Clusters or categories that are highly preferred or strongly disliked provide a third kind of information. Finally, multiple regression permits the analysis of multiple independent variables. It provides assurance that a particular physical feature is influencing a dependent variable after other constructs are taken into account. As with any analytic procedure, the results are open to interpretation by others.

The picture preference procedure was adapted for the studies that serve as a foundation for this book. All of the studies used color photographs of existing exteriors or interior spaces of assisted living buildings. A sufficient amount of the building exterior and interior space was retained so that the features under study could be viewed in context. For example, a dormer was not photographed in isolation; the surrounding roof and façade below were included as well. Exterior scenes typically focused on either main entries or an expanse of the building near the main entry. Photographs were taken from a main parking lot or street under sunny conditions with the vegetation in bloom. It was virtually impossible to photograph an entire building and at the same time exclude parking lots and retain enough detail. Interior scenes focused on entries or foyers, common living rooms, and common dining rooms. For entryways, photographs were taken of the space looking back toward the front door. For both dining rooms and living rooms, photographs were taken of the entire space from a major access point. All scenes, whether they focused on the exterior shell or interior rooms, comprised buildings that were freestanding, three stories or less, and in good condition. Interior spaces were in buildings built after 1992. Single-family houses that were designated as assisted living were not included.

A face-to-face format was used for all of the studies. Directions were read aloud, and responses were recorded by the investigator. The actual interview procedure consisted of two distinct parts: a rating scale and open-ended questions. For the first portion, participants were told that they would be looking at photographs of retirement housing whose cost and location were the same. Participants were asked to imagine they were helping a close friend or relative to select a housing arrangement and were instructed to evaluate the scenes according to a rating scale. In the second part of the interview, participants were asked to explain, in an open-ended format, why they rated certain scenes favorably or unfavorably.

More than five hundred participants, consisting of older adults and family members who could be involved in the relocation decision-making process, evaluated more than sixty different assisted living buildings that are representative of what is being designed and constructed in several regions of the United States. In the first study, seventy older adults from Michigan evaluated in terms of preference twenty-one photographs of exteriors of assisted living buildings. Results revealed that participants liked buildings that they perceived as "homelike" and disliked ones they perceived as "institutional." A pilot study, consisting of eighteen assisted living residents and eighteen family members, and a larger study, comprising one hundred assisted living residents and one hundred family members, built upon the first study. Participants from Michigan and New York evaluated the homelike character of thirty-four photographs of the exterior of assisted living buildings located in Florida, Massachusetts, and Michigan. Responses were structured through a sorting task.

Later studies focused on interior spaces. One hundred residents of assisted living in Alabama and one hundred family members completed three different sorting tasks using photographs of fourteen interior entryways, eighteen common living rooms, and eighteen common dining rooms of assisted living residences in their state. Several different rating scales were pilot tested to determine which would yield the most useful information in terms of both visual features and behavioral intent. "How comfortable would you be finding your way?" and "How inviting is this room?" were some of the questions asked. In the end, ratings of "homelike" were most effective in ascertaining participants' perceptions of what was important to them to facilitate their use of interior spaces. More detailed information about the studies can be found in Marsden and Kaplan (1999) and in Marsden (1999).

What Design Guidelines Are Provided?

The design guidelines, based on the studies just discussed, address the appearance of assisted living buildings and capture formal meanings related to shape, proportion, and scale; sensory meanings related to color, light, and texture; and symbolic meanings that arise from inferences about form and sensations (Lang, 1988). Symbolic meanings may be denotative, when people make judgments about building types (e.g., hospital or hotel) and style, or connotative, when people make appraisals about the quality and character of a building (Nasar, 1999). The design guidelines also address the instrumental use of the environment (Lang, 1987) based on inferences consumers made in the surveys from the formal, sensory, and symbolic meanings.

Thus, the design guidelines focus on the visual aspects of exteriors and interior spaces of assisted living buildings; physical features that affect the abilities of people to function effectively in exterior and interior entryways, common dining rooms, and common living rooms; and the social context. The guidelines address in depth a few of the issues important to older residents of assisted living and family members based on features that were depicted in the buildings included in the studies. Differences between both consumer groups are reconciled when dissimilar needs are identified. The guidelines also address features that should be avoided based on consumer responses.

The design guidelines do not address many other issues that are also important to the design of assisted living. Recommendations for individual resident units, hallways, outdoor areas, or back-of-house spaces such as the commercial kitchen or laundry room are not provided in this book. Please refer to Regnier (2002) for additional information based on his visits to assisted living buildings. The operational context, often intertwined with the physical environment, is not specifically addressed. Consumers were not asked about services, and staff or administrators' perspectives were not taken into account. Thus, concepts such as privacy, autonomy, and control that are documented as design goals or objectives for assisted living by other scholars are not referenced in the design guidelines in this book. In addition, urban design issues or cultural differences are not tackled, since environmental sampling and participant sampling were limited to American suburban and rural locales.

Unlike most design guidance in the assisted living literature, the design guidelines in this book were developed in relation to a strongly analytic conceptual framework that evolved from all of the studies. The guidelines address how assisted living environments *actually are* based on the way they are experienced, understood, and used by consumers as opposed to how they *should be* according to professional acceptance. Although an analytic framework shaped the design guidelines, this does not preclude possibilities for innovation. Hillier (1996) argued that theories of possibility should be explored in the creative design process after greater understanding is derived from direct study of built environments.

Some of the design guidelines in this book offer specific guidance based on empirical findings, while others inspire, rather than dictate, appropriate design responses in relation to the conceptual framework that evolved from the research. Sometimes they corroborate suggestions proposed in the past by other scholars. Other times they call into question previous recommendations. In general, all of the suggestions in this book are intended to sensitize those involved in the building development process to needs that are important to consumers. The guidelines offered are certainly not comprehensive. They are not necessarily the only solution or the "right" solution for every situation. Each guideline is still a hypothesis that may be modified in the future if put into practice and tested with additional research.

PART I   **ASSISTED LIVING**

CHAPTER 1

An Overview of the Industry

In the eighteenth and nineteenth centuries, poorhouses, poor farms, and almshouses accommodated older Americans who were without resources or family support. Nonprofit organizations, affiliated with ethnic, religious, and professional groups, built old age homes in the early 1900s to provide poor people with a way to avoid the degradation of the poorhouse. A small number of older adults who had sufficient resources rented rooms in private houses that became known as rest houses, convalescent homes, or boarding houses (ElderWeb, 2004). Decades later, in the 1980s, assisted living emerged as a derivation of board-and-care homes and as a way to keep residents out of costly nursing homes in continuing care retirement communities (CCRCs). Eventually the term *assisted living* was used by the private sector to distinguish such residences "from the mom-and-pop 'board-and-care' option that is often associated with a . . . less up-scale elderly consumer market" (Golant, 1998, p. 25), a staff with less training, and fewer personal care services (Regnier, 1999).

Assisted living became a burgeoning industry in the 1990s. At the beginning of the decade, the Assisted Living Federation of America (ALFA) was founded to advance the industry, guide providers, and enhance the quality of life for consumers (ALFA, 2001). In 1997, *Fortune* magazine identified assisted living as one of the top three promising industries (McLean, 1996). Several privately owned companies held public offerings around that time, which provided more funding sources for industry expansion.

Although it is difficult to pinpoint the number of assisted living residences in the United States because of variations in terminology and state licensing, the National Investment Conference (NIC) recently estimated that the number of assisted living residents increased 115 percent, from 362,014 to 777,801, between 1991 and 1999 (cited in Gibson, Freiman, Gregory, Kassner, Kochera, Mullen, et al., 2003). This phenomenal growth resulted in an industry that is estimated to be a $12 billion to $15 billion per year business (ALFA, 1998). At the beginning of the twenty-first century, the surging growth of assisted living faltered, affected by the downturn in the economy. In addition, inexperienced developers who misjudged market size and the dependency levels of prospective residents moved too quickly and caused overbuilding in some areas (Durand, 2001; Moore, 1998). There is now some indication that the oversupply of units has been absorbed in the market, and lending opportunities are improving (Martin, 2003; Fitzgerald, 2004). Consumer demand for assisted living is expected to continue, and the greatest growth in the older population is still to come.

Why Did Assisted Living Evolve?

Demographic Explosion

The most powerful factor fueling the evolution of assisted living in the United States is the demographic explosion of the oldest old. People age 85 years and older are the fastest-growing segment of the older population. In 2000, the U.S. Bureau of the Census (Hetzel and Smith, 2001) reported that 4.2 million people were 85 years and older, representing an increase of 38 percent since 1990 (compared to the general population growth of 13%). The population over the age of 100 is increasing rapidly as well. Between 1990 and 2000, the number of centenarians increased by 35 percent, from 37,306 to 50,454. Projections by the U.S. Census Bureau indicate that the oldest old will increase at about the same rate during the first decade of this century to 5.8 million people. This trend is expected to continue well into the future as the number of the oldest old is projected to increase 382 percent between the year 2000 and 2060 (ALFA, 2001). By 2050, it is anticipated that 19 million people, or 5 percent of the U.S. population, will be age 85 or older. Of the 19 million, there may be as many as 1 million centenarians (U.S. Administration on Aging, 2004).

With advancing age, there is a greater likelihood of disability. According to the AARP (formerly the American Association of Retired Persons) (Gibson et al., 2003), disabilities may be sensory, cognitive, physical, or emotional. Within the older population, the onset of a disability is usually slow, occurring as a chronic condition progresses. Having a disability means that a person requires assistance because of difficulty with personal care activities, known as *activities of daily living* (ADLs), or with the management of everyday activities, called *instrumental activities of daily living* (IADLs). ADLs include bathing, dressing, getting in or out of bed, using the toilet, feeding oneself, and navigating the home environment. IADLs include the ability to prepare meals, clean house, manage money, take medications, use the telephone, shop for groceries, and navigate the neighborhood outside the home. A 1999 study by the AARP found that nearly 40 percent of persons aged eighty-five and older required assistance with two or more ADLs and 12 percent needed help with IADLs in 1999 (Gibson et al., 2003).

Several social trends have affected families and their ability to support disabled older adults in their own homes. Approximately 60 percent of women over the age of twenty are in the U.S. workforce (U.S. Department of Labor Bureau of Labor Statistics, 2004), which means that they have less time to assume what has traditionally been their role as caregivers. Although the current cohort of older adults have lived most of their adult life in one locale, their adult children are more likely to have moved, resulting in a geographic separation between aging parents and adult children. In addition, the majority of older adults do not want to live with family. A survey of consumer needs found that 69 percent of older adults would prefer to move to a place that provides care services rather than live with family or friends (AARP, 1996). As a result, the formal delivery of services and specialized housing are often necessary to support the oldest old.

Consumer Demand

Consumer demand for more humane alternatives to nursing home institutionalization is another powerful factor in the evolution of assisted living. The dedication of public funds through Medicare and Medicaid fueled the growth of the nursing home industry in the 1960s and 1970s (Durand, 2001). Modeled after the hospital, the nursing home emphasized staff efficiency, which led to regimented routines, dependency, public address systems, and centralized building plans with a nurses' station in close proximity to narrow rooms along double-loaded corridors. The nursing home also emphasized safety, as reflected in stringent regulations and building codes, and the delivery of medical care to patients (Regnier, 1994). Well-documented scandals of abuse, neglect, and safety hazards have reinforced consumers' perceptions of the nursing home as a frightening and depressing place.

In the last decade, older consumers have become increasingly less willing to accept nursing home placement. Many have institutionalized a parent and are familiar with the problems that have characterized nursing homes. Adult children, often involved in the relocation decision-making process, are also reluctant to place loved ones in an institutional setting. Assisted living responded to consumer demand for a resident-centered model of care that preserves independence, autonomy, privacy, and dignity in an environment that is residential in character. As the assisted living industry expanded in the 1990s, the number of nursing home residents declined from 5.1 percent in 1990 to 4.5 percent in 2000. Among the oldest old, only 18.2 percent lived in nursing homes in 2000 compared to 24.5 percent in 1990 (Hetzel and Smith, 2001).

Economic Opportunities

The spiraling cost of skilled nursing care also affected the evolution of assisted living. A survey, conducted by Life Care Inc. for the MetLife Mature Market Institute in 2002, found that the average annual cost of nursing home placement is nearly $61,000 ($5,083 a month) compared to $25,908 a year ($2,159 a month) for assisted living. Nearly 70 percent of nursing home residents receive help from Medicaid (Gibson et al., 2003), a government program for lower-income people or those impoverished by high medical expenses. In contrast, assisted living is largely a private pay industry. Personal assets account for two-thirds of the funding used to pay for assisted living, while another 8 percent is derived from family assistance. Other sources include Supplemental Security Income (SSI) (14%), Medicaid waiver programs through individual states (9%), and long-term care insurance (2%) (National Center for Assisted Living, 2001). Thus, providers and policy makers have had a strong incentive to delay nursing home placement for older adults. At the same time, providers realized that many assisted living residents did not need twenty-four-hour skilled nursing care, and assisted living evolved to fill a gap in services between skilled nursing and independent living.

It has been repeatedly demonstrated that many older adults are willing to bear the private pay cost of assisted living. This can be partially attributed to the unprecedented growing affluence of the senior market. Nearly forty years ago, older adults were the poorest segment of the U.S. population, with a poverty rate of 35 percent (Federal Interagency Forum on Aging-Related Statistics [FIFARS], 2000). In 2001, people over the age of 65 had the lowest poverty rate, at 10.1 percent (Smith, 2003). Between 1984 and 1999, the net worth among households headed by adults aged 65 and older increased 69 percent (FIFARS, 2000). As a result, older Americans now control 70 percent of the country's assets and represent 50 percent of all discretionary income (Polyak, 2000). Even the oldest old, who live on fixed incomes and may be depleting assets, have a net worth averaging approximately $125,000 (FIFARS, 2000). As a result, providers have been responsive to consumer needs, resulting in a market-driven industry.

What Is Assisted Living?

A Confusing Industry

To be responsive to the needs of local stakeholders, individual states, rather than the federal government, have assumed responsibility for the development, management, and operation of assisted living. As a result, assisted living reflects a wide range of providers, staffing, services, acuity levels of residents, costs, and physical design attributes. Assisted living is even known by a multitude of names, such as personal care homes or residential care facilities, because of different licensing categories in each state. Some have argued that such diversity provides consumers with a great deal of choice when selecting assisted living residences (Hyde, 2001). Others think that diversity leads to confusion among consumers and providers about the purposes of assisted living (Namazi and Chafetz, 2001).

In 2001, the U.S. Senate Special Committee on Aging asked a broad-based coalition, called the Assisted Living Workgroup (ALW), to develop a specific, consumer-friendly definition of assisted living as part of a larger report of recommendations to improve the quality of care in residences nationwide. After eighteen months, the ALW, consisting of forty-nine organizations representing providers, consumers, health care professionals, and regulatory agencies, was unable to craft a definition that was fully supported by at least two-thirds of the participating organizations. Organizations disagreed over several aspects of the definition, including the disclosure of specific services in a resident's contract, the definition of health-related services, the requirement for privately occupied units, and the establishment, in an attempt to decrease costs, of levels of licensing categories based on the acuity level of residents (Assisted Living Workgroup, 2003).

While it may be impossible or even undesirable to develop a common definition of assisted living, several elements have been agreed upon. Assisted living is state regulated and monitored. Assisted living offers a range of personal and health care services, delivered by professionally trained providers, to meet scheduled and unscheduled needs on a twenty-four-hour basis. Assisted living offers housing that is residential in character and appearance. The delivery of supportive services and housing is based on a philosophy that addresses the needs and preferences of residents; maximizes residents' independence, dignity, privacy, autonomy, and decision making; and involves family members. When assisted living is viewed as an alternative to the continuum of care rather than as an option between independent living and skilled nursing, aging in place is also a philosophical goal of assisted living.

Consumer-centered Services

More and more states are adopting an assisted living philosophy that organizes the delivery of services around the resident. Terms such as privacy, independence, dignity, decision making, and autonomy are reflected in state policies (Mollica, 2001). To put the philosophy into practice, some states have developed a negotiated-risk process that respects a resident's preference for care despite the risk to the resident that may be involved. Mollica (2001) provides an example related to bathing. A resident has the decision-making control to undress privately, get into a tub, and bathe on his or her own, even if a staff or family member believes the resident is at risk of falling. Once the risk is documented and the resident assumes responsibility for the decision, the provider may not be liable. This is a challenging process, since it is difficult to define risks and determine what liabilities can be waived (Zimmerman, Sloane, and Eckert, 2001b).

According to Mollica (2001), specific services that may be offered in assisted living are determined by move-in and move-out criteria for each state related to health and care conditions and the ambulation and cognitive needs of residents. In general, the level of services that may be offered and the acuity level of residents who may be served in assisted living have been increasing. States that support aging in place allow more extensive services, such as skilled nursing, under certain conditions for a limited time. Such services are contracted through home health care agencies or, to a lesser degree, offered on site. Regulations typically identify who can administer nursing services directly or through delegation to unlicensed staff (Golant, 1999). Regulations also specify whether medication can be administered and the extent to which assistance with administration is permissible. In addition, state rules require agreements or contracts that provide residents with an understanding of available services, fees, resident rights and responsibilities, and move-out criteria. The National Center for Assisted Living (NCAL) has assembled a report that summarizes the regulation of assisted living for each state (Bentley, Sabo, and Waye, 2003).

Despite the wide range of services that may be offered in assisted living due to variation in regulations, recent national surveys indicate that certain services are commonly offered (ALFA, 2000; NCAL, 2001; NIC, 1998). These include assistance with ADLs, help with the timing and coordination of medications, congregate meals and snacks, housekeeping, laundry and linen service, transportation to shopping and doctors' offices, social and recreational activities, exercise classes, and an emergency response system. Other services offered to a lesser degree, depending on state regulations and commitments to aging-in-place, include incontinence management, administration of medication, health services such as physical therapy and podiatry, health assessments, and skilled nursing. Depending on the rules of individual residences, smoking in designated areas, drinking of alcoholic beverages, small resident-owned pets, and overnight guests may be permitted.

| Residential Housing | In addition to consumer-centered services, assisted living offers housing. The design and construction of assisted living residences are influenced by regulatory oversight that varies from state to state. States that have based their policies on the philosophical goal of privacy require single occupancy apartments with baths (Mollica, 2001). Other states permit shared bedrooms and bathrooms and vary in the number of residents that can share these spaces. States that espouse the goal of autonomy require unit kitchenettes or equipment to store and prepare food (Mollica, 2001). Many states also use the terms *homelike* or *residential* in their philosophy statements. These terms are linked to the presence or absence of features that enhance autonomy and privacy. Other physical plant requirements that vary include the amount of square footage for residential units and environmental provisions for residents with dementia (Bentley, Sabo, and Waye, 2003). |

In addition to meeting state licensing requirements, assisted living residences must comply with local building codes, fire safety regulations, federal laws, and zoning ordinances to safeguard public health, safety, and welfare. In 2000, the international building code (IBC), a comprehensive set of national codes, was published to facilitate consistent code enforcement and compliance throughout the country. In the past, three different building codes were used in various regions of the United States, which led to diverse interpretations. Many states and municipalities have been adopting the IBC since its publication. Under the new national code, assisted living residences with six to sixteen occupants are now classified as residential (R-4), while residences with more than sixteen occupants are still classified as institutional (I-1). Other changes include the requirements for fire extinguishing and detection systems based on building height and allowable building area, more relaxed exiting requirements, and more restrictive firewall protections. Local fire codes also specify how exits should be secured and require emergency and evacuation plans. Specific federal requirements that must be considered include the Americans with Disabilities Act of 1990, which requires buildings to be accessible to persons with physical and certain mental disabilities. Zoning laws typically specify separate land uses for buildings with institutional classifications, which has segregated some assisted living residences from the rest of the community. The public is often concerned about the effect of assisted living residences and nursing homes on property values, traffic congestion, and community resources, even though no studies have shown that senior housing affects the value of single-family housing (Arenson, 1998).

Despite the overlapping restrictions imposed by state regulations, building codes, and fire safety and zoning laws, assisted living is still regulated less stringently than are nursing homes. Nursing homes, in fact, are the second most heavily regulated buildings after nuclear power plants. Assisted living regulations that are less strict and more flexible have allowed designers to experiment with residential character and to offer a variety of solutions to consumers. As a result, assisted living has assumed many physical forms. Some residences are remodeled large private homes, schools, or hotels. Many are freestanding structures, ranging from one story to multiple stories, specifically designed to incorporate the assisted living philosophy. Others are wings of nursing homes, independent living or congregate apartments, or part of continuing care retirement communities. Regardless of the arrangement of buildings, the individual units vary from semiprivate rooms to studio and one- and two-bedroom apartments. According to recent national surveys, two-thirds of assisted living residences are purpose-built, freestanding buildings (NCAL, 2001; ALFA, 2000) with an average height of 1.8 stories (NIC, 1998). The average number of units is 66.5 (ALFA, 2001), which is an increase over previous estimates of approximately fifty. According to ALFA (2000), the majority of units are studios (61%) with an average of 300 square feet, followed by one-bedrooms (21.9%) averaging 515 square feet, semiprivate rooms (12.6%) averaging 315 square feet, and two-bedroom apartments (2.5%) averaging 727 square feet. Approximately one-quarter of assisted living buildings include a dedicated wing or floor for residents with dementia (ALFA, 2000).

Who Does Assisted Living Serve?

Frail Older Adults

Assisted living serves a frailer population than was initially intended. Recent national studies have indicated that the average age of assisted living residents is approximately eighty-four (ALFA, 2001; NIC, 1998). Disability is prevalent because of cognitive, emotional, physical, and sensory impairments. According to NCAL (2001), 23 percent of residents have been diagnosed with Alzheimer's disease, with 19 percent in the early to middle stages of the disease. Another 29 percent suffer from other forms of mostly mild dementia. In addition, about one-quarter of assisted living residents suffer from depression. With respect to sensory changes, about one-third have a significant hearing impairment, and a similar proportion have a visual impairment that cannot be corrected with glasses (Hyde, 2001). The most common medical conditions among residents include bladder incontinence (33%), heart disease (28%), bowel incontinence (18%), osteoporosis (16%), and diabetes (13%) (NCAL, 2001).

Because of disability, the average assisted living resident needs help with 2.25 to 2.8 ADLs (NCAL, 2001; ALFA, 2001), compared with 3.8 ADLs for nursing home residents, as reported by the Health Care Financing Administration (cited in NCAL, 2001). Approximately one-fifth of assisted living residents do not require any assistance with ADLs. According to NCAL (2001), 72 percent require at least some help with bathing, and 57 percent require at least some help with dressing. There is a need for a lesser degree of assistance with toileting (41%), getting in and out of bed (36%), and eating (23%). Many residents are also dependent or require assistance with IADLs. In particular, more than three-quarters of assisted living residents need at least some assistance with medication use and money management. About one-half need at least some help with using the telephone. Travel inside and outside the assisted living residence is affected by the resident's mobility. ALFA (2000) found that 59 percent of residents are ambulatory, 41 percent require the assistance of a mobility aid such as a wheelchair, walker, or cane, and less than 1 percent are nonambulatory or bedridden.

A Homogeneous Group

Approximately three-quarters of assisted living residents are women (ALFA, 2001), which is not surprising, considering the greater longevity of women. There were only forty-one men aged 85 years and older for every one hundred women aged 85 years and older in 2001 (Hetzel and Smith, 2001). The majority of residents are also single. Seventy-three percent of residents are widowed, 10 percent are married, 9 percent were never married, and 9 percent are divorced or separated (Hyde, 2001). This is also not surprising, since most older women are widowed and are prompted to seek care outside the home. In contrast, most older men are married and often receive care from their spouse at home. In 2002, only 11.8 percent of women compared to 57.6 percent of men aged 85 years and older were married with a spouse present in the home (Smith, 2003). Most residents of assisted living buildings are not only widowed females; they are also white. Again, this is not surprising, since diversity is less evident among the older population than among the younger population. Eighty-seven percent of those aged 85 years and older compared to 69 percent of the total population were non-Hispanic white in 2002 (Smith, 2003). In addition, there are cultural differences between certain racial groups regarding the use of long-term care. For example, Mutran, Sudha, Reed, Menon, and Desai (2001) found that older African Americans in North Carolina prefer family care more than do older whites, but this is partially due to a perceived lack of acceptable options.

What is surprising is that assisted living residents may not be as wealthy as previously assumed. Income is difficult to identify in surveys because of the sensitive nature of the subject, and available reports differ on average income levels. One study, conducted by Price Waterhouse Coopers (ALFA, 1998), indicated that the national average income of assisted living residents was $30,831 and that their average net worth was $153,000 in 1997. Another study, which was conducted by the National Investment Conference around the same time (1998), found that nearly two-thirds of assisted living residents had an annual income below $25,000 and an average net worth of less than $100,000. The average annual cost of assisted living, however, was approximately $24,000 when the studies were conducted, and 86 percent of assisted living residents did not receive public or private assistance in addition to their income (NIC, 1998). This suggests that assisted living residents are liquidating their assets to cover assisted living fees. Since the average length of stay in an assisted living residence is reported as 24.5 months (ALFA, 2000), 30.8 months (NIC, 1998), and 36 months (NCAL, 2001), the net worth of residents may be just about enough to sustain their residency.

Family Members

For many older adults, the relocation decision-making process involves family input. NIC (1998) found that someone other than the older adult initiates the relocation process in more than half of the cases. According to Claritas, Inc., a national demographic firm, family members are the strongest source of referral for an assisted living residence, followed by media advertisements and hospitals (Tinsley and Warren, 1999). The most influential family members are typically daughters between the ages of forty-five and fifty-five (Dixon, Parshall, Pratt, Solinger, and Young, 2001). In 28 percent of cases, an older adult does not even visit the prospective assisted living residence before move-in and instead relies on family feedback (NIC, 1998). As a result, the marketing of assisted living residences is often directed at family members, even though older adults pay for assisted living and occupy the residence on a daily basis.

After an older adult relocates to an assisted living residence, family involvement, one of the philosophical goals of assisted living, is encouraged through caregiving partnerships. Family members may be able to bridge communication gaps between residents and staff (particularly if the resident is suffering from some dementia), ask pertinent questions, and provide emotional support. Visitation is encouraged. In some instances, special events, volunteer programs, shared activities, shared meals, or overnight stays have been organized to draw family members to assisted living. According to a national study conducted by NIC in 1998, 95 percent of residents received at least one visit from a family member or friend in the preceding thirty days. This is possible largely because of the family's proximity to the assisted living residence. As a result of the move, more than three-quarters of older adults have family within twenty miles of the residence (Tinsley and Warren, 1999).

CHAPTER 2

Design Resources for Assisted Living

Design is generally understood as a process during which concepts and mental images are generated in response to a program, client, site, and budget as well as building codes and regulations. Concepts and images are externalized and communicated through two- and three-dimensional representations that are eventually articulated as working drawings for building construction. In a series of cycles, designers continuously appraise tentative representations against an array of information, backtrack, and then revise earlier decisions as they move toward a solution (Zeisel, 1984). This process is not easily traced because designers do not completely adhere to a set of prescribed rules (Groat and Wang, 2002).

Hasell and King (in press) proposed that four forms of knowledge, arranged along a continuum of increasing validity and rigor, guide design decision making. The first form, consisting of subjective hunches, speculations, or intuitions that are believed to be valid, is the weakest and most commonly used. Other forms of knowledge along the continuum are needed to supplement and strengthen the designer's intuitions. The second form, proposition, refers to the logical and empirical use of the existing literature to provide grounding for hypotheses. Persuasion is a third form of knowledge shaped by objective research findings from either quantitative or qualitative empirical studies. Findings "persuade" or convincingly provide evidence indicating a relationship between the environment and human behavior based on associations among variables. Finally, objective research findings that are causal, measurable, and repeatable make up the most precise form of knowledge, which is called demonstration. This fourth form of knowledge is the most difficult to attain, and few examples exist in the environment and behavior literature.

What Knowledge Sources Are Available to Guide the Design of Assisted Living?

Award Competitions

Each year award competitions sponsored by organizations such as the American Association of Homes and Services for the Aging, the American Institute of Architects, the Assisted Living Federation of America, the Center for Health Design, and the Society for the Advancement of Gerontological Environments recognize outstanding assisted living projects. Architects, designers, and providers are encouraged to submit entries consisting of building images, drawings, and brief program statements. Reviewers or judges primarily comprise practicing architects and interior designers, researchers with a design background, and administrators. Occasionally other judges include a regulator, resident, or family member. The criteria used to evaluate the submissions are often written in an intentionally vague way to encourage a wide range of interpretations among the design solutions. Images, descriptions, and reviewers' comments highlighting the positive aspects of each project are documented in books such as the *Design for Aging Review* series published by the American Institute of Architects Press or trade journals such as *Contract Magazine* and *Nursing Homes Long Term Care Management.* In addition, projects are presented at professional conference sessions or are part of a conference exhibition.

Practitioners assume that these projects are "best practice" examples and apply lessons learned from award-winning designs to future projects. The evaluation process for award competitions, however, like design juries in architecture and interior design programs, is highly subjective and unpredictable (Anthony, 1991; Nasar, 1999). As a result, information that is gleaned from competitions typically consists of subjective speculations that fall within Hasell and King's first form of knowledge. Scholars have suggested that architecture firms should document the role of research in the design process (Carpman and Grant, 1993) and include an evaluation of a project with input from users and decision makers after occupancy (Nasar, 1999; Sommer, 1983; Verderber and Refuerzo, 1999) as part of the award competition submission. This would help strengthen the information that is presented to practitioners in trade journals and at conferences.

Design Guides

Design guides translate relevant information about the domain of environment and aging into design implications that are useful for practitioners. Many design guides in the field specifically focus on the needs of people with dementia in the context of a wide range of settings, including nursing homes, special care units, assisted living, group homes, and day care centers (Calkins, 1988; Brawley, 1997; Briller, Proffitt, Perez, and Calkins, 2001; Briller, Proffitt, Perez, Calkins, and Marsden, 2001; Cohen and Weisman, 1991; Marsden, Briller, Calkins, and Proffitt, 2001; Perez, Proffitt, and Calkins, 2001; Zeisel, 1999). These books of design guidance mostly consist of hypotheses grounded in the literature or the professional and personal experiences of expert scholars. Hypotheses are normative propositions, as in Hasell and King's second form of knowledge, for how the environment may, rather than will, affect human well-being. Empirical research is often needed to validate or modify hypotheses to prevent ineffective ones from guiding standard practice. For example, Cohen and Day (1993) systematically gathered information about twenty diverse settings, identified by experts, through a standardized questionnaire and face-to-face interviews with staff and administrators. When the collected data for each case study was critically analyzed in relation to hypothesized design principles developed by Cohen and Weisman (1991), some of the assumptions underlying the principles were affirmed while others were called into question.

Unlike the design guides that focus on dementia care settings, the few that address assisted living for the most part are based on the systematic collection of data from projects identified by experts (Brummett, 1997; Regnier, 1994, 2002; Regnier, Hamilton, and Yatabe, 1995). The assisted living guides are therefore more persuasive and fall within Hasell and King's third form of knowledge. For example, Brummett (1997) developed design considerations for homelike character based upon a literature review and information gathered at 16 sites though open-ended observations and interviews with forty-three residents and twenty-two caregivers. The design guides by Regnier (1994) and Regnier, Hamilton, and Yatabe (1995) are based on an initial review of 230 projects as well as site visits to 25 projects in the United States and 100 projects in Scandinavia and Holland. Each site visit entailed a 70-question interview, presumably with administrators, and a 144-item architectural checklist. Design suggestions are structured around themes that emerged from comparisons across site visits and are followed by case studies of exemplary projects that integrate the recommendations. The methodological basis for Regnier's (2002) most recent design guide is less clear. He indicated that the ideas for his book are derived from consulting experiences, conference presentations, classroom seminars, discussions with colleagues and friends, site visits, interviews with several hundred people in five different countries, and postoccupancy evaluations. This suggests that his latest design guide may be based on a blending of propositions and persuasive findings.

Benchmarking Studies

Benchmarking studies provide architects and designers with objective standards of measurement that they can comparatively analyze and apply to the design of assisted living buildings. This type of information is most closely associated with Hasell and King's third form of knowledge. The Assisted Living Federation of America (ALFA) (2000), National Investment Conference (NIC) (1998), and National Center for Assisted Living (NCAL) (2001) have conducted several national surveys that provide descriptive statistics related to the physical characteristics of existing buildings. The average square footage of buildings, number of floors, number of units, square footage of units, building construction cost per square foot, number of private units, and typical unit features are some of the benchmarks provided. Other statistics that might influence design decision making, such as staffing patterns and common activities, are also noted.

The ALFA study consisted of a self-administered questionnaire that was mailed to providers who are members of ALFA. Responses included 373 residences for the 2000 survey and 307 residences for the 2001 supplement. Four different self-administered questionnaires focusing on physical plant issues, resident characteristics, services, and staffing made up the NCAL (2001) study. A total of 318 providers completed the questionnaire regarding the physical plant. In contrast, the NIC (1998) study included questionnaire responses from 178 providers of assisted living buildings constructed in the last fifteen years as well as 1,023 interviews with residents or their caregivers.

On a much smaller scale, Moore (1999) made comparisons across ten projects, identified by experts, reflecting a range of architecture in assisted living. Both the providers and the architects of each project provided information related to characteristics of the building, organization, and residents through self-administered questionnaires. Six experts in disparate geographical areas then used a five-point scale to evaluate each of the projects in relation to twenty-eight design objectives identified from the literature. Some examples of the design objectives are the provision of a social kitchen and outdoor space, residential exterior imagery, and coherent organizational zoning.

Empirical Research

Empirical research can be used to validate or modify hypotheses presented in design guides, to evaluate a range of environmental interventions and strategies, and to validate design practices. Depending on the methodological rigor used, empirical research findings may "persuade" through an association of variables, as in Hasell and King's third form of knowledge, or "demonstrate" that there is a cause-and-effect relationship between variables, as in Hasell and King's fourth form of knowledge. Empirical research is usually documented in academic journals or as research reports. Unlike the information presented in design guides, empirical findings and scholarly journals are often difficult for designers to understand and access, which has hampered research utilization among designers.

Within the field of environment and aging, most of the empirical research that has been documented in scholarly journals is persuasive. The majority of studies address design for older people with dementia. Gitlin, Liebman, and Winter (2003), Day and Calkins (2002), and Day, Carreon, and Stump (2000) all offer comprehensive and critical reviews of the burgeoning research in this subset of the field. They state that the majority of studies include small sample sizes at single building sites, rarely attempt to include firsthand experiences of residents with dementia, and exclude comparison groups or randomization with control groups. These limitations have yielded tentative rather than conclusive findings. Furthermore, most of the research focusing on design for dementia has been conducted in the context of nursing homes. Thus, it is unclear whether the reviewed research is applicable to other settings, such as assisted living.

Empirical research that has specifically addressed the design of assisted living is scant. A few studies have focused on design issues based on data gathered from residents, family members, staff, or administrators. Frank (1999, 2002) conducted eighteen months of ethnographic fieldwork, primarily consisting of in-depth interviews with residents, administrators, and staff at two assisted living sites. She found that there is a distinct difference between homelike environments and a home. Marsden and Kaplan (1999) and Marsden (1999) conducted a series of studies, the basis for the design recommendations in this book, which examined older persons' and family members' perceptions of assisted living architecture and design. Mitchell and Kemp (2000) and Sikorska (1999) found that smaller buildings are associated with higher levels of satisfaction based on interviews with residents. Greene, Hawes, Wood, and Woodsong (1998) conducted focus groups with family members of assisted living residents and found that safety and access to safe outdoor areas are primary concerns in relation to quality. In addition, Zavotka and Teaford (1997) interviewed residents to investigate frequency of use of and preferences for interior common spaces. Other notable examples that address the assisted living environment in some capacity are documented as unpublished theses and dissertations. These include Barry (1999), Elrod (2002), Levin (2001), Rylan (1995), and Turnbull (2001).

A few scholars have conducted postoccupancy evaluations (POEs) of assisted living residences. POEs systematically assess building performance and human response to a single building using a variety of methods after occupancy. Information generated by a POE can be used to improve the project being evaluated or to inform design decision making in a future project (Zimring, 2002). Several POEs of assisted living are included in a book edited by Schwarz and Brent (1999a). For example, Hoglund and Ledewitz (1999) identified key findings from a three-year evaluation of Woodside Place, an assisted living residence for thirty-six people with dementia, and discussed the application of findings to the design of other facilities. The evaluation, conducted by Perkins Eastman Architects (Silverman, Ricci, Saxton, Ledewitz, McAllister, and Keane, 1996), measured the influence of organizational, programmatic, and environmental factors on resident health and social experience through interviews, rating scales, and observation of residents. Although not as detailed and systematic, Cinelli (1999) discussed the evaluation of an assisted living project based on interviews with administrators and some residents. Other architecture firms such as Dorsky Hodgson have indicated that they evaluate their projects a year after construction (Bonvissuto, 2003). Although their study findings have been presented at professional conferences, a literature review did not reveal published research findings.

The largest and most comprehensive empirical research on residential care and assisted living is documented in a book edited by Zimmerman, Sloane, and Eckert (2001a). One aspect of the study (Sloane, Zimmerman, and Walsh, 2001) included direct observation of the physical environment of a stratified sample of 193 assisted living residences and 40 nursing homes in four states. Trained environmental researchers completed the Therapeutic Environment Screening Survey for Residential Care (TESS-RC), a standardized instrument that measures concrete objective characteristics of the environment, in a thirty- to forty-five-minute systematic walk-through of each building. Questionnaires completed by administrators provided additional data. Based on descriptive findings, the authors developed design strategies for assisted living in conjunction with several goals that are believed to enhance quality of life. As the authors noted, however, the measures of the TESS-RC are based on the opinions and advice of experts in the field of aging and environment and have not been tested empirically in relation to resident outcomes.

Why Is There a Dearth of Rigorous Knowledge?

Explosive Growth

Amid the explosive growth of assisted living in the 1990s, few developers, providers, architects, and designers had time to assess the success of existing assisted living projects before proceeding with new construction. Since the period of design conceptualization through construction and occupancy is approximately two years, it is impossible to evaluate innovative design ideas in a timely fashion. "Not surprisingly, many facilities are designed not on the basis of solid empirical research, but simply on what the competition is doing" (Calkins, 2001a, p. 45).

Vischer (2001) noted that architecture and design firms ordinarily do not commit the resources for a postoccupancy evaluation through fees, the construction bid, or the operating budget of the building. Many firms also do not have in-house staff with the necessary skills to direct studies. Even though evaluation results might inform the design of future projects, possible negative feedback may be viewed by providers as requiring costly changes to an existing building design or by architects as criticizing professional performance. At the same time, few retirement communities are willing to commit resources to develop research centers that would evaluate buildings (Day and Calkins, 2002).

As a relatively new industry that has grown considerably in a short time, assisted living is still evolving. With little consistency in nomenclature, licensing, regulations, level of care, and design attributes, it is difficult to conduct research at multiple residences in different states and to make meaningful comparisons. This may be why most of the research in the field of environment and aging has been conducted in nursing homes. Nursing homes are more clearly defined, building designs vary less because of more stringent regulations, and residents' lives are much more controlled, which facilitates comparison across individuals (Day and Calkins, 2002).

Diverse Interpretations of Research

The Association of Collegiate Schools of Architecture (ACSA), American Institute of Architects (AIA), and Architectural Research Centers Consortium (ARCC) established the Initiative for Architectural Research (IAR) in 1997 to promote and facilitate research in architecture and to strengthen the role of knowledge-based design decision making. In 2001, the IAR sponsored a panel session with representatives from various disciplines as part of the ACSA annual meeting in an attempt to define architectural research and its relationship to design. Although the panel asserted that a definition is essential, there was little consensus (Nowakowski, 2001). Not surprisingly, *research* continues to be a term that is used broadly in the design fields. It has been described as a "google" search on the Internet, a casual walk through a building, the creation of sketches, or any activity that involves information gathering. In a recent study, Wang (2003) critically assessed current architectural research by reviewing 253 papers from four ACSA conferences.

He found that more than half of the published papers were subjective speculations that lacked robustness.

In their comprehensive book of architectural research methods, Groat and Wang (2002) carefully made a distinction between design and research, stating that "generative figural production is a different mode of inquiry from analytical research" (p. 118). "Research activity tends to be defined by propositional components: strategy, tactic, hypotheses, 'the literature,' measuring instruments, data, and so forth. . . . The generative design process, on the other hand, emerges from other workings within human reason, workings that cannot be fully explained in a propositional way" (p. 105). Groat and Wang also provided a definition of architectural research, drawing upon the work of Snyder (1984). They noted that architectural research is a systematic inquiry involving the conscious collection, categorization, analysis, and presentation of information in relation to objectives or research questions. The systematic inquiry is directed toward the creation of knowledge, which often occurs in small increments through various means. While most architectural research focuses on the physical outcomes of design, research on the process and practice of design is possible, too.

A Challenging Construct

Assisted living is a confusing industry due to wide variations in licensing, services, and built form; similarly, the field of aging and environment lacks a standard definition of the environment (Gitlin, Liebman, and Winter, 2003). Some researchers have viewed the environment primarily in physical terms, referring to site planning considerations, the appearance and form of the building from the outside, and the appearance, volume, configuration, and planning of interior spaces. The majority of studies in the field have looked at one or two discrete variables in isolation without accounting for other potentially meaningful variables. In contrast, a few studies have looked at several variables in the context of the entire physical environment. For example, to study the effect of a floor pattern on human behavior, the size and purpose of the space with the floor pattern, the amount of floor area covered by furnishings, the presence of natural lighting, and the type of artificial lighting must also be taken into account. A more holistic approach to the physical environment assumes that many variables work together, which makes it difficult to control the design features under investigation. However, this approach more closely reflects "the reality of living in a multidimensional environment" (Gitlin, Liebman, and Winter, 2003, p. 92).

It has also been suggested that the physical environment is part of a larger system consisting of people, the social context, and the organizational context (Cohen and Weisman, 1991). For example, the physical environment may provide opportunities for resident and family interaction through the arrangement of spaces and furnishings, but policies and programs associated with the organizational context must encourage family visitation and involvement in order to facilitate interaction. More recently, Calkins (2001b) proposed an integrated model of place in which historical, cultural, and societal forces also shape the environment. Similarly, Corcoran and Gitlin (1991), in earlier studies, conceptualized the dementia care environment as four interrelated hierarchical layers consisting of physical objects, tasks that use objects, the organization and composition of social groups, and culture or beliefs that shape the way in which care is provided. In a somewhat different vein, Schwarz (1999) conceptualized the assisted living environment as a place type, which takes into account the way the building is used, the physical properties of the building, the processes that control the way the building is developed, and associational and symbolic meanings that contribute to how buildings are understood. The multidimensionality of all of these models adds greater complexity to the measurement of the environment.

PART II   **HUMANISTIC DESIGN**

CHAPTER 3

Design Guided by Research-based Consumer Input

The Johnson Wax building was designed and constructed as the administrative headquarters for S. C. Johnson & Sons Inc. in Racine, Wisconsin, in the 1930s. Several decades later, an article in the *Wall Street Journal* noted: "To the art historians, it is a masterpiece. The sleek, three-story building, designed down to the doorknobs by famed architect Frank Lloyd Wright, has been described not only as this country's 'greatest piece of 20th century architecture' but 'possibly the most profound work of art that America has ever produced.' Then again, the historians never worked there" (Schellhardt, 1997). The 160 employees who work in the office building on a daily basis must deal with the ever-shifting play of light and shadows, mice that get trapped in the glass tubing that replaced conventional windows along the perimeter of the great work room, acoustical problems that make it impossible to conduct meetings or use speaker phones, and three-legged chairs that cause serious back problems (Schellhardt, 1997).

The literature and popular press are filled with numerous examples of critically acclaimed buildings that are designed in ways that do not support people's well-being. This has largely been attributed to the efforts of well-meaning designers who are apparently unaware of user needs. In assisted living, there has been a movement toward the delivery of services to residents based on needs and wishes they have articulated. There has been little attempt, however, to do the same with the design of the physical environment. Humanistic design is based on consumer input. Older people who occupy assisted living buildings and family members who periodically visit should have a say about the design of the environment they use. Architecture is public, and designers have an obligation to consider the needs and preferences of consumers. This is possible when consumers are asked about their needs and perceptions of environments in the context of scientific research.

How Can Consumers Provide Input Related to Design?

Research from Consumers Applied by Designers

Consumers, such as older adults and family members, can provide input about the design of assisted living as part of a scientific study. In this traditional research approach, researchers systematically collect information directly from a representative sample of consumers to understand how they perceive and use their environment or perceive and would use other environments under investigation. Familiar with the language of both research and design, researchers then analyze the collected data, report results, and translate findings into design implications or guidelines that are generalizable. If the information is understandable and accessible, designers who are receptive to research can use the recommendations to improve an existing building or to inform the design of future buildings. In either case, there is a separation between the designer and the consumer, with the designer indirectly addressing the consumer's point of view. There is also a division between research and application.

Researchers can collect information from consumers with one-on-one, structured or unstructured interviews, focus groups, or survey questionnaires. These methods, which rely on statements directly from consumers, require much less inference on the part of the researcher than do other methods (Lawton, 2001). For example, direct observation of consumers requires the researcher to draw inferences about desirable environmental features from nonverbal expressions, locations, and behaviors of consumers. Similarly, expert judgments are required for direct observation of certain aspects of the physical environment (Lawton, 2001). Some researchers have used visual information in conjunction with interviews, focus groups, and questionnaires. Visuals have been used to understand how consumers experience their physical environment. To study legibility, Lynch (1960) asked residents to sketch maps of their city; Cooper Marcus (1995) requested homeowners to draw a sketch that reflected their feelings about their current home. In other instances, visuals such as models, photographs, or drawings have represented proposed or existing environments and provided consumers with a range of alternatives in a format that they can easily understand. This makes it possible to study a variety of existing buildings in scattered locations without having to obtain responses on site (Hershberger, 1988).

Several strategies have been recommended to facilitate the acquisition of information from cognitively intact older consumers. First, a face-to-face format, with questions read aloud and responses recorded by the researcher, is considered ideal regardless of the instrument type (Lawton, 1987). Advantages include the possibility of moderating speech patterns to aid the hearing impaired, circumventing dexterity problems encountered by those completing questionnaires, ensuring that instructions are understood and information is accurately recorded, tailoring the pace of the procedure according to the abilities of the participant, and establishing a rapport to facilitate cooperation. In addition, some older adults view the face-to-face format as a pleasant visit. Nevertheless, older adults may attempt to engage the researcher in conversation, which can extend the already lengthy time frame required for the face-to-face format. The researcher's approach and appearance may also influence responses. Second, a simple question-and-answer approach is the easiest for older adults, but novel tasks that are accompanied by careful explanation and practice may be possible (Lawton, 1987). Marsden (1999) found that the sorting task is an effective way to engage older adults and reduce the monotony associated with most surveys. In his studies, older adults were asked to sort photographs into piles marked with bold, large type, based on a five-point rating scale. Sekulski, Jones, and Pastalan (1999) developed and used an assessment game with older adults to elicit their daily life activities in the context of their environment. Third, visual material makes it easier for older adults to respond to environments they have never experienced. Large, clear visuals can be handled to allow older adults to view material closely at a pace they determine. Fourth, questions can be framed in a way that makes it acceptable for older adults to provide negative responses. If older adults are asked to evaluate environments in a way that directly challenges their competence, they are less likely to identify problems that can be rectified (Lawton, 1987).

It is frequently assumed that it is not feasible to seek input about environmental issues from cognitively impaired older adults. Many older adults with dementia are immediately excluded from studies that involve interviews, focus groups, or questionnaires. It is also assumed that surrogates of cognitively impaired consumers can accurately provide information on their behalf. Lavizzo-Mourey, Zinn, and Taylor (1992), however, found low correlations between ratings of surrogates and of cognitively intact nursing home residents with respect to care and the environment. Similarly, Berlowitz, Du, Kazis, and Lewis (1995) concluded that nurses had little insight into cognitively intact nursing home residents' quality of life. It is likely that it is even more difficult for surrogates to provide information from the perspective of the cognitively impaired. Chaudhury argued that the quality of research on design and dementia would be greatly enhanced if firsthand experiences of older adults with early to middle stages of dementia were elicited (cited in Day and Calkins, 2002). Uman, Hocevar, Urman, Young, Hirsch, and Kohler (2000) recognized that it is possible to interview older adults with dementia when interviewers are carefully trained, consumers are appropriately selected, and techniques adequately compensate for reduced cognition. In one study that focused on the environment, Zeisel (1999) conducted a focus group with five people with dementia to understand how they define home. Participants were able to provide responses both verbally and pictorially.

Research and Design with Consumers

A less common way that consumers can provide input about the design of assisted living is through action research. Unlike traditional research designs, this approach integrates research, design, and participation and facilitates collaboration between researchers, designers, and consumers to effect social change in a particular context (Sanoff, 2000). In a predesign phase, the researcher, acting as facilitator, works with the designer and local consumers to define the parameters of a design project for a particular community. Formal research techniques, such as the ones discussed in the previous section, are used in a cogenerative learning process to create a shared vision and to identify important goals (Greenwood and Levin, 1998). Once an overall understanding has been achieved, action is taken to develop the desired physical environment. Older adults and family members may formulate design ideas and share them with the designer and researcher. In contrast, the designer and the researcher may develop conceptual schemes and present alternatives to the consumers for review. Research techniques that consider the methodological needs of older consumers, as discussed previously, can be used to systematize the review process. As all the stakeholders move toward a final solution through mutual learning and negotiation, the results of actions are interpreted and compared to the goals that were identified at the beginning of the process.

Action research provides several advantages that are not possible with traditional approaches to research on environment and behavior. First, research knowledge is generated to address the problems of a specific design project and is applied during the design process to resolve those problems. This is possible because research and design activities are performed simultaneously rather than sequentially, which makes the link between research and practice stronger. Second, action research provides a framework for the use of environmental programming and its integration into the design process. The predesign phase gives designers reliable information and helps to minimize the time that is usually wasted by designers attempting to second-guess consumers' needs (Sanoff, 2000). Third, action research directly addresses the perspective of consumers by treating them as coresearchers and codesigners. Consumers are empowered to share in the decision making for a specific project and thus actively shape the environment they will use.

Why Is Consumer Input Important?

Different Perceptions between Designers and Consumers

The designer's and the consumer's ways of seeing are dissimilar. Several studies have repeatedly demonstrated that architects both conceptualize and evaluate environments differently than do nonarchitects, leading to disparities in perceptions and preferences (Devlin, 1990; Devlin and Nasar, 1989; Groat, 1982; Hershberger and Cass, 1988; Hubbard, 1994; Nasar, 1989; Purcell, 1995; Rodriguez, 1994; Stamps, 1991). Such differences have been attributed to design education and professional experience. In schools of architecture and interior design, for example, students spend a great deal of time studying the physical environment, engaging in design, and criticizing buildings. As a result, they develop a different set of constructs and values for understanding and evaluating the built environment (Groat, 1982). Wilson (1996) found that this difference is most pronounced in the last two years of education and concluded that it "appears that architects are 'taught what to like'" (p. 40), and this is often at odds with what the general public prefers.

Some scholars have argued that architects know they see the environment differently than consumers do and reject popular preferences because they disagree with them (Gans, 1974; Saint, 1983; Wolfe, 1981). On several occasions, famous architect Philip Johnson has stated that popular tastes are "vulgar" (Nasar, 1999). Le Corbusier commented that the public required reeducation, suggesting that architects can change consumers' preferences to ones that are favorably viewed by designers (Nasar, 1999). Research has shown, however, that the public's preferences for the built environment remain stable over time (Stamps,

1997). Other scholars have noted that architects are concerned with consumer needs but unknowingly see the environment differently and simply misjudge popular preferences (Brown and Gifford, 2001; Nasar, 1989). Brown and Gifford (2001) asked architects to predict a typical nonarchitect's global impression of forty-two different buildings. Some architects were able to predict public responses better than other architects, and this may be linked to less design experience. Architects who were unsuccessful with predictions were unable to exchange their conceptual criteria with criteria used by the public to make judgments, which strongly suggests that greater contact between designers and consumers could help minimize differences in perceptions and preferences.

Shared Consumer Needs

A lack of formal design training does not interfere with a consumer's ability to make meaningful evaluations of environments. "There is a tendency to regard expert opinion as always more reliable and correct. For many aspects of the environment, the experts are the people who know most about using it—the users" (Sanoff, 2000, p. 87). Consumers make judgments about environments based on perceptions and patterns of use that educated design experts do not share. This is particularly true as people age and become more sensitive to and reliant on the environment. How an eighty-five-year-old woman, for example, navigates an assisted living dining room is probably very different from how a forty-year-old architect will use the space. Certain design features will be more important to the eighty-five-year-old person than to the architect. Consumers may not always be able to specify desirable features or to articulate reasons behind their evaluations, but researchers can extract underlying perceptions through statistical analyses.

A common misconception is that "there is no accounting for people's tastes." This suggests that it is fruitless to elicit judgments about the environment from a specific consumer group, such as older adults, because each person's taste in that group is idiosyncratic and random. The research literature does not support this concern. Although individual differences exist, humans have much in common because of their shared physical world, biology, evolutionary history, and culture (Nasar, 1999). This has led to strong consistencies in the way people interpret the environment and shared categories of information that people find important in the environment. Over the last several decades, researchers have identified common human needs that are central to the design of natural settings (as summarized in Kaplan and Kaplan, 1995; Kaplan, Kaplan, and Ryan, 1998) and the design of the built environment (as summarized in Nasar, 1999). These findings have shown remarkable stability.

Consumer Well-being

It is well established that there is a reciprocal interdependence between human behavior and the environment. It is also well established that environmental design is an important component of long-term care and can influence the psychological and physical well-being of residents and the quality of care by staff. When consumer input is taken into account, it is more likely that the environment will work better for the people who use the environment and will enhance interactions between people. This can lead to greater consumer satisfaction, which, in turn, may lead to a better maintained physical environment, greater consumer enthusiasm and acceptability for a building, and financial savings in terms of occupancy levels and potential retrofits (Becker, 1977). Zeisel (2003) pointed out that, if developers, owners, operators, residents, family members, and staff were aware of the benefits of specially designed environments, such as those that incorporate the consumer perspective, they might demand them.

Why Is Consumer Input Lacking?

The Widening Gap between Designers and Consumers

In primitive societies each member built his or her own house according to a uniform model developed by the larger group. This model was adjusted over time to satisfy climatic, physical, and maintenance requirements (Rapoport, 1969). The same person was the designer, builder, client, and user and knew exactly what was needed. According to Rapoport (1969), the development of specialized building trades in pre-industrial times led to a differentiation between builders and clients (who were also users). Both groups shared and respected the cultural model of housing and worked together to introduce individual variations. The client/user remained an active participant in the design process, and craftspeople offered more detailed knowledge related to construction, form, layout, and the site. Vernacular design traditions emerged as a result.

Since the Industrial Revolution, housing has been designed and built in different ways. In some instances, a private client secures the services of an architect to design a house that the client will eventually occupy. The client and the architect are usually from the same social background, share similar values, and have little trouble communicating. The needs of the client are simply conveyed through the criticism of design schemes. The architect then hires contractors to build the house. For the majority of Americans, houses are designed and built by architects, developers, speculative builders, and contractors with whom the prospective homeowners will never collaborate. Although this results in a gap between designers and the people who will occupy the houses, selective buying and sensitivity to market conditions can help narrow the gap to some extent (Zeisel, 1984). In this scenario, the eventual users of the building are actually consumers.

The emergence of other housing options, such as assisted living, that are more complex and that accommodate larger numbers of people has led to a distinction between intermediate consumers who pay for and determine the design of the building and end consumers who use the building (Verderber and Refuerzo, 2003). Intermediate consumers of assisted living typically include corporations, nonprofit organizations, administrators, and developers, while staff, residents, and family members are the end consumers. Even though the end consumers are directly affected by the design of the building, they have no control over the design process and little or no control over the environment after occupancy. The intermediate consumers hold all the power (Verderber and Refuerzo, 2003).

The Insular Education of Designers and Consumers

Graduates of design programs bring their educational values into practice, which perpetuates the isolation of designers from the public they are intended to serve. First, the design studio, the focus of architecture and interior design education, physically and socially separates students from university life. Students are cloistered together in the same building for long hours and rarely interact with future consumers across campus. Second, many design instructors discourage collaboration with the larger community to minimize design constraints. Project descriptions typically include hypothetical consumers or do not include consumers at all. Students usually work alone during the design process, with feedback from the "master" instructor, and marginalize the experiences of consumers. Evaluations by outside practitioners address artistic innovation and intuitive form-making rather than the responsiveness of the building to consumers. Third, with the exception of design-build and service learning studios, most projects are driven by theory rather than real everyday experiences. Few architecture and interior design programs prepare students for social challenges such as our aging population. As a result, students begin to believe that they know what is best for consumers and use themselves as a model for what all other humans need. In a study by Tzamir and Churchman (1989), 168 students primarily relied on their own personal experiences during the design process even though they reported that they had addressed user needs a great deal.

For the most part, the public is not even aware that architects and designers are educated in a way that breeds isolation. Frank (2002), an anthropologist by training, noted that her earliest examinations of housing environments for older adults led her to "a shocking conclusion: no one was asking residents about *their* needs or perceptions of their environment. Many designers, policy makers, and planners were simply acting on the residents' behalf, and creating residential environments that *they* believed would be functional for residents" (p. ix). Frank's dismay can be attributed to the insular education of consumers. Architecture and interior design courses are not part of the liberal education of high school and university students. In addition, design electives are not usually open to nonmajors on college campuses. The environment, however, is an important part of everyone's world. Consumers who are interested are exposed to a narrow portion of the design field through travel, critical discourses focusing on famous buildings, or neighborhood walking tours focusing on historic architecture. Television networks and programs that concentrate on home remodeling and decorating may provide greater exposure, but they may also fuel stereotypes and mislead consumers about what design actually entails.

Many are struggling to bring designers and consumers together through changes in architectural education. Recent studies stress a need for greater consumer sensitivity in design, interdisciplinary collaboration, and social responsibility (American Institute of Architecture Students [AIAS], 2002; Anthony, 1991; Boyer and Mitgang, 1996; Cuff, 1991; Fisher, 2000). Similar needs have been identified abroad (Nicol and Pilling, 2000). Such ideas, however, are antithetical to the outdated pedagogical philosophies of the École des Beaux Arts in Paris and the Bauhaus in Germany. These former European academies largely shaped the first architectural programs in the United States in the late 1800s and continue to strongly influence the design studio today (Association of Collegiate Schools of Architecture [ACSA], 2004).

At the same time, some are struggling to bring consumers and designers together through public education. Zeisel (2003) described how one company markets the environmental design of its assisted living residences to consumers through mission statements, brochures, in-person presentations to families, and reprints of journal articles that are viewed as objective endorsements. He also noted that environmental design should be marketed to the larger community through lectures at professional meetings and conferences, professional training seminars, and media outlets to generate even more exposure. With greater education, consumer demand for design input may evolve.

Consumer Recruitment Challenges

Seeking consumer input about the environment is particularly challenging with older adults, since many are reluctant to participate in research. Some cite poor health, sensory deficits, or fatigue. Others are suspicious and uncertain as to what participation involves, fear that participation will reveal their ignorance or cognitive impairment, equate participation with test anxiety, are uncertain about the benefits of participation, do not want to sign a consent form, or believe that participation will not lead to change. Many think they have little to contribute to environmental design in particular and society in general. "What can you possibly learn from me?" or "I don't have anything interesting to tell you, my life wasn't that exciting" are common reasons for refusal (Frank, 2002, p. 18). When older consumers are residents of assisted living, it is necessary to seek the permission of administrators and family members to recruit them for a study. Some administrators may be hesitant about the close scrutiny of their residents by outsiders or may not want to invest the time to alert family members. Residents may fear reprisal from management for disclosing something negative and may refuse participation as a result.

Seeking input from family members also raises recruitment challenges. Many investigators seek the help of administrators of assisted living. Administrators are usually not able to share contact information for family members and must be willing to devote the time to get in touch with relatives on the researcher's behalf. It may be possible to recruit family members directly through residents. However, many residents do not have family close by or do not want to impose on relatives' visits or time. Other investigators may try to identify family members in the community. Since a sampling frame (a list of the population from which the sample is drawn) for adult children with aging parents does not exist, investigators usually target support groups for relatives with aging parents or rely on personal connections and professional contacts. Such a reliance on convenience sampling is widespread in gerontological research (Camp, West, and Poon, 1989) and affects the ability to generalize results.

A few researchers have examined ways to improve recruitment among older adults and family members. When older adults are residents of assisted living, professional experience suggests that it is useful to meet with administrators in person, sometimes without making an appointment, to explain the purpose of the research and to request cooperation. If permission is granted, a familiar staff person can introduce the researcher to potential participants to ease apprehensions. Harris and Dyson (2001), in their research in nursing, indicated that the researcher can find out information about potential participants from staff members beforehand and then use that information to relate to the older adults. They also suggested that the researcher should approach the potential participant at an optimal time and avoid mealtimes, activity sessions, or moments after an unpleasant incident. It is advantageous to meet in a location deemed comfortable by the participant. When an initial rapport has been established, it is important to explain the study in a concise and clear way. In many instances, it is necessary to assure older adults that their memory will not be tested (unless that is part of the actual study), that participation merely entails their opinion, and that participation will not require them to purchase anything. Many must also be convinced that they have something worthwhile to share.

CHAPTER 4

Research-based Conceptual Framework

Most design guidance has been shaped by theories that are strongly normative and weakly analytic (Hillier, 1996). In other words, architectural theories have been easily used to generate designs based on professional acceptance of how environments should be, but they have been weak in predicting what designs will be like when built. This is particularly true in the assisted living literature. "There are few descriptive positive theories consisting of statements and assertions that describe and explain the reality of assisted living and that are capable of extension to predictions of future reality" (Schwarz and Brent, 1999b, p. 304).

The empirical research that serves as a basis for this book generated a strongly analytic framework that is concerned with how assisted living environments actually are based on the way they are experienced, understood, and used by consumers. The framework is not intended to explain through causal relationships. Rather, it is conceptual and links some aspects of human behavior in relation to some characteristics of the current assisted living environment. It is intended to inform the normative design guidelines that follow in the next portion of the book. Because of the research, the guidelines provide a more finely tuned domain for the designer to work in and a more dependable sense of how a building will perform when it is built.

The conceptual framework consists of six salient constructs, identified from the consumer perspective, that are central to the design of humane assisted living environments: familiar housing cues, protective enclosure, caring cues, human scale, usability, and naturalness. The constructs address the appearance of assisted living buildings and capture formal meanings related to shape, proportion, and scale; sensory meanings related to color, light, and texture; and symbolic meanings that arise from inferences about form and sensations (Lang, 1988). Based on messages that are read from formal, sensory, and symbolic meanings by consumers, the conceptual framework also addresses the instrumental use of the assisted living environment (Lang, 1987). McCracken's (1989) work on homeyness served as a foundation for an earlier version of the conceptual framework (Marsden, 2001).

The conceptual framework for humanistic design touches upon many of the concepts that have been identified in the conceptual frameworks of other scholars in the environment and aging field. These include the concern for safety, security, and orientation and the desire for social interaction, familiarity in the environment, sensory stimulation, a homelike appearance, and a connection to the family (Regnier, 2002).

Since the studies that serve as a foundation for this book did not address resident dwelling units or the operational context, the conceptual framework for humanistic design does not address the concepts of privacy, autonomy, and control that are also commonly noted in other conceptual frameworks for assisted living environments and services (Regnier, 2002).

Familiar Housing Cues

To determine whether an environment is familiar, people relate current stimulation to memories of past experiences with environments. These experiences are stored as internal representations. Each representation is "a summary from a series of nonidentical experiences with a given object" (Kaplan and Kaplan, 1982, p. 26). In other words, this internal structure is not a copy or template of an environment; rather it is an economical unit of knowledge consisting of the salient features of an environment. Familiarity results when characteristics of an environment have been frequently encountered before and there is a fit between current stimulation and an existing internal representation. This can lead to a positive affective response. When current stimulation is largely discrepant from an internal representation, an environment is experienced as unfamiliar, and such an experience can evoke a negative affective response (Purcell and Nasar, 1992). Nasar (1999) reviewed several empirical studies of the built environment confirming that people, with the exception of artists and architects, prefer low levels of novelty in the environment.

The single-family detached house is a familiar living arrangement for many older adults. More than three-quarters of Americans over the age of forty-five occupy a house (AARP, 2000) and identify with this cultural icon over a lifetime. In contrast, assisted living is an unfamiliar housing type. The integration of memory-jogging symbols, spatial and furniture arrangements, purpose-specific rooms, and terminology associated with the house may help to make assisted living more familiar to older adults (Marsden, Briller, et al., 2001). For example, familiar housing symbols in the Midwest include pitched roofs, porches, and fireplaces. Familiar spatial arrangements comprise a front door that leads to more public and formal areas of the house such as a living room or dining room, a back door that leads to a kitchen or family room for informal gatherings, and a transitional hallway that leads to private bedrooms. A familiar furniture arrangement includes chairs at right angles with an end table and lamp in between. When a space is used for its intended purpose, its familiar symbols and arrangements are reinforced. For instance, a space that includes a table set with napkins, dishes, and silverware suggests that eating is an appropriate activity. Spaces that are identified with language such as "living room" as opposed to "lounge" are also more familiar. In addition, some diversity is a familiar cue. Many houses include windows of varying sizes and shapes rather than uniform windows across a façade. Similarly, the same chair is rarely used in a dining room, living room, and bedroom.

Protective Enclosure

Enclosure has to do with "the dream of being sheltered and protected—the need to be inside *something* that motivates us all. Being inside a cave, inside a room, under a canopy, within a great domed enclosure, behind a fence, in an arena, on a balcony, or on a porch, all are conditions of enclosure which carry specific connotations" (Moore, Allen, and Lyndon, 1974, p. 143). This need for enclosure in order to feel safe and protected is certainly not new and can be traced historically. "Many early buildings hugged the earth like a bear cub's den, designed for protection against tornadoes as well as excesses of heat or cold. Ranch houses were designed for protection against enemies and the sun, with air circulation in mind; porches were added for sitting outside and as a center for observation and conviviality. Many vernacular houses represent a safe place, almost a fortress, a reflection of a basic tribal memory of the need for security, a need that modern man, beset by different enemies, feels as strongly as his forebears" (Kavanaugh, 1983, p. 13).

In the built environment, protective enclosure is probably most associated with the roof. Frank Lloyd Wright (1954) often provided a ground-hugging "broad protecting roof shelter" (p. 33) with large projecting eaves over the whole building to give the dwelling the "essential look" of shelter (p. 16). The roof overhangs also protected the walls, another enclosing element that affords protection. Rapoport (1969) asserted that the pitched roof as opposed to the flat roof is symbolic of shelter, while Rand (cited in Alexander, Ishikawa, Silverstein, Jacobson, Fiksdahl-King, and Angel, 1977) found that people still see the pitched roof as a powerful symbol of shelter even after being exposed to the flat roofs of the Modern movement during the twentieth century. Boudon discovered that the modernist houses built by Le Corbusier in Pessac, France, were completely transformed by a succession of occupants. In many cases flat roofs were replaced with pitched ones and open terraces were covered (cited in Jacobson, Silverstein, and Winslow, 2002). Alexander et al. (1977) stated that a roof must not only be large and visible but also include living quarters within its volume. "The roof itself only shelters if it contains, embraces, covers, surrounds the process of living" (p. 570).

Other features reinforce the notion of protection through layers of enclosure, which help to separate public and private zones. Trees, lawns, shrubbery, and fences provide enclosure at the outermost public layer. Ivy or other vegetation on exterior walls offers another level of protection, while narrow, small-paned windows, as opposed to big areas of clear glass, solidify the walls. Balconies and porches are transitional zones between the public street and the building envelope and offer semipublic areas from which to view the surrounding environment. Within the building, bookcases, artwork, and furnishings that line walls offer a final layer of protection for the private interior. Spaces can also provide a feeling of enclosure. The building form itself can create sheltered outdoor spaces. Balconies that are recessed or are covered with roofs provide a greater sense of protection than those that project beyond the building. Similarly, porches with covered roofs, railings, and solid walls behind suggest protection. Well-defined interior spaces with low ceilings afford enclosure, while alcoves, nooks, window seats, and bay windows imply personal enclosure. Enclosure may provide a general sense of support, assurance, and protection for vulnerable older adults.

Caring Cues

A physical environment may express care directly through the act of building, "as in the meticulous gingerbread details in the little houses at Oak Bluff on Martha's Vineyard in Massachusetts" (Moore and Allen, 1976, p. 139). Care, however, is probably most associated with maintaining or tending a place (Moore, Allen, and Lyndon, 1974). When landscaping is neat, fences are freshly painted, and details like window boxes or shutters are given attention, care is evident (Nassauer, 1995). Empirical study of the built environment indicates that upkeep increases preference, while dilapidation is often cited as a reason for disliking an environment (Nasar, 1997). Maintaining a place also suggests that there is a human presence. A person has been to that place and returns often (Nassauer, 1995). Signs of occupancy such as drawn curtains, open windows, tended plants, and information desks also suggest human presence. Human presence, as demonstrated through occupancy and attention to details and maintenance, implies that support is nearby if needed. This may provide assurance for older persons who are likely to feel vulnerable if they are dealing with age-related losses and impairments.

An environment that is welcoming also communicates care. In this sense, a building should metaphorically open itself up, welcoming the observer and inviting entry in the process. A glazed entry door, for example, can provide a glimpse of what is inside a building, alleviating any fears of the unknown, and can allow the person approaching the building and those within to prepare for a reception. Similarly, window views from the interior of a building to an outdoor activity may elicit curiosity and foster participation. In addition, an environment can be welcoming when shared spaces and furniture arrangements create a comfortable atmosphere, bring people together, and encourage social exchange. A welcoming environment is very important to older adults, who are more likely to feel isolated and unsure as a result of age-related impairments.

Human Scale

What exactly is meant by human scale? This is not always entirely clear, just as the concept of scale itself is often referenced in a variety of ways. "We talk, for instance, of a large-scale housing development, and we usually mean just that it is big. In a different context, we say that an architectural drawing has a scale, meaning that so many units of measure on the drawing represent so many units of measure in the actual building. Then there are super scale, miniature scale, monumental scale, and—perhaps the most talked about of all—human scale" (Moore and Allen, 1976, p. 17). One theme common to the various uses of the term *scale* is that the size of something is being compared to something else. For example, "a large-scale development is large in comparison to an average housing development" (p. 17). That is not to say that scale is the same thing as size. Rather, "scale is *relative* size" (p. 18). Another commonality is that scale involves expectations based on past experiences (Orr, 1985). For instance, "super scale usually means that something is much bigger than we might have expected, miniature scale that it is much smaller" (Moore and Allen, 1976, pp. 17–18). Most things have a usual size, which gives us a sense of how we should relate to them. A brick that is oversized, for example, will be inconsistent with our expectations and may seem disturbing as a result.

Human scale, then, suggests that something relates to the size of a human. Frank Lloyd Wright (1954) indicated that the body could serve as a measuring device in relation to the house. He stated that "human scale was true building scale" and used five feet, eight and one-half inches, his own height, "to fix every proportion of a dwelling or of anything in it" (p. 16). For instance, he eliminated "useless heights" or "empty grandeur" by lowering ceiling heights and roofs. The latter was accomplished by relocating servant quarters, which were typically located in attic spaces in the earlier part of the twentieth century, to rooms adjacent to the kitchen on the ground floor. In addition to human height, Orr (1985) indicated that the spread of a human's arms, the length of a stride, and the size of a grip with one's hand are sources of human scale. A doorknob that can be easily grasped, especially if placed at a comfortable height from the ground, a brick that can be easily held with one hand, steps that have wide enough treads and risers within a certain range, and a doorway that is wide enough to pass through are examples. We cannot use these features easily unless they are related to the dimensions of the human body.

With respect to the overall building, Orr (1985) asserted that greater attention to elements of a building that are large in relation to the body rather than to smaller features, such as doors, stair railings, or window panes, tends to make a building appear monumental. In contrast, greater attention to smaller parts helps to create a feeling of intimacy or diminutiveness (Orr, 1985). The distance of the front entrance approach, the expansiveness of the site, the overall building form and height, the volume of interior spaces, the distances between spaces, and the level of ornamentation on the outside and inside of a building also affect human scale. Human scale is particularly important when dealing with a housing type such as assisted living, which is larger than the single-family house, and a group such as the elderly, who are typically more vulnerable than the general population. A building that emphasizes human scale is likely to be more manageable both visually and as a place to use physically.

Usability

Usability is a measure of how well users can access and effectively negotiate an environment. It is also the degree to which an environment enables users to complete tasks and activities. Environments that are usable help sustain people's physical independence. When people are able to function on their own, their sense of personal worth and self-confidence may be enhanced. In addition, they are more likely to believe that they have control over their environment. If a building does not support patterns of use for intended users, deleterious effects are possible.

Usability is particularly important for older people. Older adults experience the environment through sensory modalities that have been altered by aging. In particular, a decrease in visual acuity, an increase in sensitivity to glare, a reduced ability to adapt to changing light levels, low vision due to common eye diseases, a decline in hearing, and reduced touch sensitivity may affect older peoples' abilities to interpret the environment and respond appropriately. As a result, environmental signals must be stronger and simultaneously appeal to multiple senses for older adults to perceive them (Briller, Proffitt, Perez, and Calkins, 2001). According to Briller, Proffitt, Perez, Calkins, and Marsden (2001), several other physical changes may influence older peoples' abilities to access and use the environment. For example, a reduction in muscle mass and elasticity, bone loss, and the stiffening of joints in the musculoskeletal system reduce strength and flexibility, affecting mobility and dexterity. Cardiopulmonary changes such as a decreased lung capacity, cardiovascular disorders including hypertension, and foot conditions such as corns and toe and nail deformities can also affect mobility. In addition, cognitive changes that make it difficult for older adults to remember recent events, recognize places, things, or people, and execute a sequence of actions may adversely affect functional abilities. Specific features such as orientation cues, spatial and furniture arrangements, and floor, wall, and ceiling finishes that support the remaining abilities of older adults help to make the environment more usable.

Naturalness

Naturalness can be interpreted as close association to the natural environment through landscape elements, views to the outdoors, and the authentic use of building materials, color, light, and plants. Nassauer (1995) reviewed studies in the literature on landscape perception that suggest that some landscape elements communicate naturalness. These studies have repeatedly identified elements such as vegetation, especially canopy trees, and water. Kaplan and Kaplan (1978, 1982), in their studies of natural environments, suggested that certain landscape elements, such as water and trees, are considered desirable and enhance preference. The Kaplans contend that such preferred "contents" are linked to our evolutionary history and are interpreted as elements needed for survival. Nature itself is also a preferred content, and research has indicated that natural environments are preferred over both urban and residential environments (Kaplan, Kaplan, and Wendt, 1972). Research has also shown that views of nature from building windows provide opportunities for mental restoration (Kaplan, 2001), enhance postoperative recovery and health (Ulrich, 1984, 1995; Verderber, 1986), and positively affect satisfaction with neighborhoods (Kaplan, 1985; Talbot and Kaplan, 1991) and jobs (Kaplan, 1993).

Building materials can be considered modified elements of nature. Wood, for instance, was once alive. Although it doesn't continue to grow once it is cut down, it continues to remind us of its natural origins through its appearance, texture, and sometimes even its smell. The connection between materials and nature was particularly strong at one time. "The materials from which a building was made came virtually from the site itself: stone was cut from local quarries and timber from neighbouring forests; brick and tiles were baked in clay from nearby pits. There was a strong link between the artifact and the earth from which it grew that was not just economic, but deeply satisfying at a psychic level too" (Materiality and Resistance, 1994, p. 4). Color was also linked to nature. Often this was true because color is integral to specific building materials, such as red brick, and their weathering qualities. In addition, color was tied to specific regions and sites. "One of the most popular in New England—then and now—is red, which was applied on the exteriors of barns and houses to help absorb solar heat. In the days before paint was manufactured, New Englanders created a mixture of rust (scraped from nails and fences), skim milk, and lime that coated the wood like a varnish" (Kemp, 1987, p. 25).

This connection among materials, color, and nature was weakened "in the Industrial Revolution, when materials that had been common in one part of a country could be transported to another as whims of production and economics dictated" (Materiality and Resistance, 1994, p. 4). More traditional materials such as wood, brick, mud, straw, and plaster were tied to the site, processed and put together by hand, but buildings now are usually mass produced—built of factory-made, factory-finished materials. The connection between materials and nature was further weakened by the advent of modern materials and construction techniques. For instance, modern materials such as reinforced concrete, steel, plastic, imitation stone, and wood laminates are usually not perceived as "natural." "Steel is hard, cold, bearing the impress of the hard, powerful industrial machines that rolled or pressed it; plastic has something of the alien molecular technology of which it is made, standing outside the realm of life and, like reinforced concrete, bound by no visible structural rules" (Day, 1990, p. 113). These modern materials are also often used in a deceptive way—vinyl siding replicating wood—which tends to corrupt the nature of materials. As a result, authenticity is questionable and modern materials tend to "look as fake and hollow as they sound when you tap them" (Day, 1990, p. 116). Frewald (1989) indicated that natural building materials such as fieldstone and wood, as opposed to synthetic materials or those that appear manufactured, enhance preference largely because they serve as connections to the natural environment.

PART III   **DESIGN GUIDELINES**

CHAPTER 5

BUILDING EXTERIORS

First impressions are very important. The front façade of a building, the main entry, and the surrounding landscape greatly affect people's initial perceptions of an assisted living environment. Based on curbside appeal, prospective consumers may enter a site or just drive away. They may move closer to the building or turn around. They may be drawn to the front door, the focal point of the building exterior, or discouraged from entering based on inferences they have made about the interior spaces. Older adults who occupy an assisted living building on a daily basis and family members who periodically visit are not only concerned about the exterior appearance and the meanings that are conveyed by the façade and surrounding landscape; they are also concerned with the potential utility of the environment. For instance, certain aspects of the exterior entry may encourage consumers to sit and visit or may discourage socialization if deemed uncomfortable.

Based on the assisted living buildings that were depicted in the studies that serve as a foundation for this book, exterior features that are important to consumers as well as attributes that should be avoided were identified and translated into design guidelines. The design guidelines that follow take into account formal, sensory, and symbolic meanings as well as patterns of use that are pertinent to the humane design of the exteriors of assisted living buildings.

For enhanced understanding, the guidelines are discussed in relation to the conceptual framework explained in the previous chapter. Each construct of the framework can be considered a design goal. The highlighted statements under each design goal are more specific design recommendations. Each design recommendation is then described and supported by findings from the studies. Occasionally, empirical research from other scholars is referenced to provide additional support. Interpretation is facilitated by presenting the design guidelines in tandem with photographs of existing assisted living buildings, the majority of which were used during data collection for the studies. Each photograph is referenced throughout the chapter, since each image may provide examples of both favorable and unfavorable features. Figure captions summarize these features.

When a guideline relates to more than one construct of the framework, it is linked with the construct that offers the clearest explanation. References to other constructs are mentioned or included in parentheses. Although the construct of usability is referenced throughout, it is not included as a separate section in this chapter. Usability is a substantial portion of the following chapters, which deal with interior spaces.

Familiar Housing Cues

Reconsider the Placement of the Porte-cochere. The porte-cochere, an open-sided roof structure that projects out over the driveway, is a common entry feature on the front of assisted living buildings. It not only provides a sheltered drop-off area between the car and the front door but also draws attention to the entry and creates visual drama and depth. Both older adults and family members, however, indisputably considered this entry feature oversized and an unfamiliar housing cue that communicates institutionalization (fig. 5.1). The long drive and vehicular approach of the porte-cochere suggested to many consumers that a bellhop would be waiting at the entrance to take their luggage. The width of the driveway and signage indicating clearance heights also suggested that the entry could accommodate a truck, a funeral hearse, or an ambulance and evoked images of other building types, such as hospitals and funeral homes. Even porte-cocheres that include parallel drive-by lanes for emergency vehicles and are smaller in scale as a result were rated very unfavorably (fig. 5.2).

In certain regions of the country where snow and ice are a problem, a sheltered driveway is desirable for older adults when they leave the building for social outings or doctors' visits. Designers perhaps should reconsider the placement of the porte-cochere. A porte-cochere that is an extension of the front façade as opposed to an imposing front addition is a more familiar housing pattern. Many examples are evident in older homes that were designed to accommodate carriages and vehicles, as shown in figure 5.3. In addition, the porte-cochere can be used on the side of the building. Two principal façades, one with a porte-cochere and the other with a familiar housing entry, can create separate vehicular and pedestrian access points.

Explore Variations of the Portico for Pedestrian Covered Walkways. In milder climates, some shelter along a covered walkway from a driveway

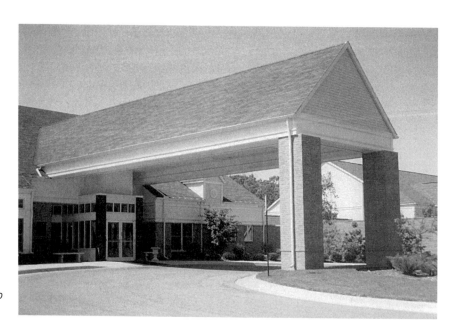

Figure 5.1. The porte-cochere is often an oversized and unfamiliar housing cue that communicates institutionalization to consumers.

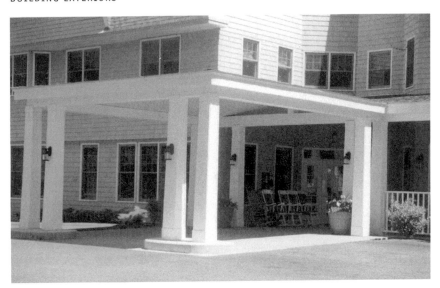

Figure 5.2. *A smaller porte-cochere with a parallel drive-by lane is an unfamiliar housing cue.*

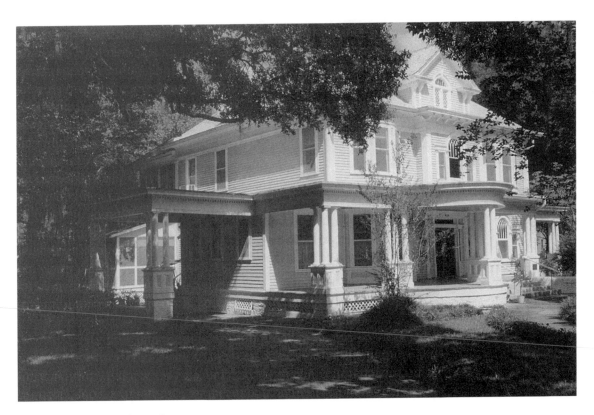

Figure 5.3. *Many older houses incorporate a porte-cochere that is an extension of the front façade rather than an imposing front addition.*

to the front door, as opposed to a porte-cochere, may be all that is needed for protective enclosure. However, the design of the pedestrian covered walkway affects its desirability. Older adults tended to favor some small-scale shelter over the entry, as with porticos and pedestrian covered walkways. Even when a sheltered walkway included an unfamiliar housing cue such as a canopy, older adults still rated this somewhat favorably (fig. 5.4). When the scale became too large, however, the need for familiar housing cues became more important to older adults

49

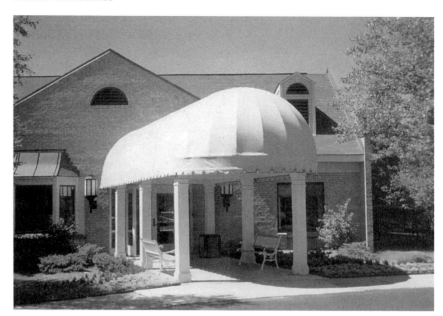

Figure 5.4. *Even though a canopy is an unfamiliar housing cue, older adults viewed it more favorably than did family members because it provides shelter over the walkway to the entry.*

than actual sheltered covering. Family members, in contrast, viewed all types of sheltered entries, other than smaller porticos, negatively. The canopy implied to many family members that they might be attending a wedding or a funeral. Familiar housing cues were more important to family members than was sheltered covering.

To reconcile differences between older adults and family members in terms of shelter, human scale, and familiar cues, designers should explore variations of the portico along pedestrian walkways. A portico is a covered entrance that often uses columns to support a roof with a pediment. The assisted living building in figure 5.5, for example, includes a portico that projects several feet beyond the building edge to the driveway to provide shelter. Positioning the door close to the driveway helps to reduce the distance that needs to be traversed and prevents the extended portico from becoming an oversized and unfamiliar housing cue. There are many other ways that porticos can be adapted to provide shelter over a walkway in a manner familiar to consumers.

Embrace the Porch. For both older adults and family members, the porch was a comforting cue of familiarity in assisted living buildings. The porch, a sheltered entryway that is partially open or enclosed along the outside of a building, can be used as a familiar cue on the front façade in a variety of ways. It can include floor-to-ceiling windows, half-walls with screens above, or railings with an open framework. Although some porches merely include supporting columns, some protective enclosure is recommended at the edge. The protective enclosure can serve as a physical support that older adults can lean on as they navigate the porch area. This enhances usability. The porch can also be inset if a portion of the external walls under the main roof of the building is omitted or can be attached to the building with its own roof and walls or

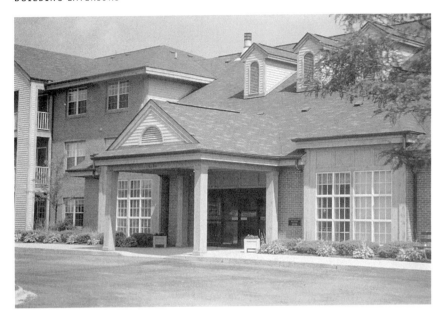

Figure 5.5. *Porticos that project beyond the building edge can provide shelter over a short walkway in a manner that is more familiar than a canopy.*

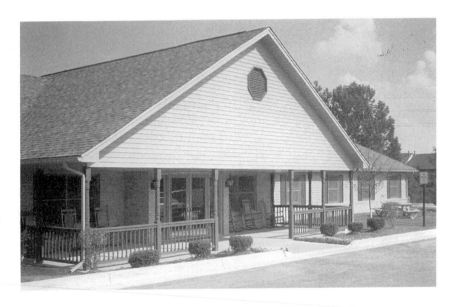

Figure 5.6. *A porch can function as a pedestrian covered walkway when it is located close to the driveway and is level with the ground. Signs of human occupancy, such as seating and picnic tables, communicate caring, and one-story porches provide human scale.*

railings. It can cover a portion of a façade, extend across an entire façade, or wrap around multiple façades. It can also function as a pedestrian covered walkway if it is located close to the driveway and is level with the ground, as shown in figure 5.6. Although consumers noted that this porch was awkwardly proportioned, they still rated it favorably. When a porch is raised several feet above grade, it is desirable to incorporate a ramp in the porch design by using the same architectural language, as shown in figure 5.7. Usability is enhanced as a result.

Reference Exterior Features of the Single-Family House. In addition to porches and porticos, older adults favorably viewed certain features of the façade that evoked images of the single-family house. Family members more broadly preferred features that reminded them of the house

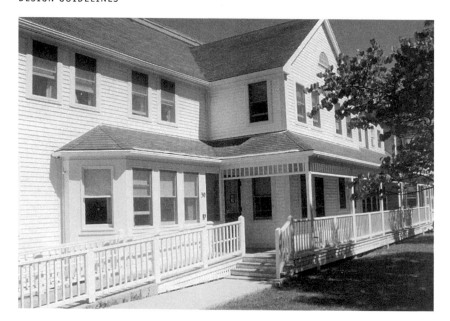

Figure 5.7. *When a porch is raised several feet above grade, a ramp and railing using the same architectural language as the porch enhance the usability of the entry in a contextually compatible way.*

as well as apartment buildings, townhouses, or condominiums. Features that were desired by both groups of consumers are recommended for assisted living buildings. In particular, front gables, side gables, and cross gables drew positive responses and helped to reinforce the sloped roof. The pitch of the roof did not seem to matter to consumers as long as the roof was evident from the ground level. Window shutters were desired and easily identified if painted a color that contrasted with the façade. The manicured front lawn has been a powerful status symbol for most Americans since the era of suburban expansion after World War II. Consumers rated the front lawn of assisted living buildings, a feature of naturalness, favorably. Even more mundane, utilitarian features, such as gutters and downspouts, were well received. In contrast, unfamiliar cues that should be avoided include metal and glass front doors, flat roofs, and freestanding flagpoles in the middle of the lawn.

Vary Windows and Balconies. The size, spacing, and number of windows and balconies along the façade are often the basis for initial inferences about interior units. Windows and balconies that are all the same size and shape and are spaced uniformly imply that all units are the same and that all occupants, in turn, are viewed similarly. This evoked images of institutionalization among older adults and family members. Thus, some diversity is a familiar cue. Many single-family houses include windows and balconies of varying sizes and shapes to accommodate different functions within. Research also indicates that moderate diversity in the built environment is preferred (Nasar, 1999). Thus, it is advisable to consider windows and balconies that vary. Such variation, when included in individual resident units that face the front of the building, offers residents a choice when selecting a unit for occupancy. Units that differ in any capacity, however, sometimes present marketing chal-

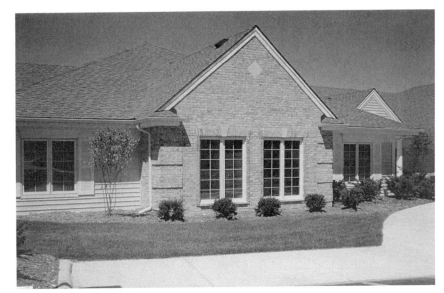

Figure 5.8. *Housing cues familiar to consumers include a sloped roof, gables, window shutters, gutters and downspouts, and windows of different sizes and shapes. Details, such as window muntins, lintels, and quoins, suggest careful attention to the act of building and provide human scale. The variety of rooflines and a combination of building materials help to reduce the perceived massiveness of the façade.*

lenges. It may then be more advisable to incorporate a combination of common areas and units toward the front of the building so that windows can vary in relation to different spaces. Figure 5.8 depicts an assisted living building that includes familiar housing cues such as a sloped roof, gable, window shutters, a gutter and downspout, and windows of different sizes.

Protective Enclosure

Accentuate Edges with Layers of Enclosure. The exterior entry can provide protection from inclement weather as described previously. Other features of the façade and surrounding landscape can reinforce the notion of protection through layers of enclosure. Fences at the outermost edge of the property help to reinforce the site itself and tie together all the landscaping and building features they surround. Unlike tall, solid fences that do not permit views out or in, picket and wrought iron fences provide enclosure in an unimposing way and were favored by consumers. Front lawns, entries such as attached porches, and individual balconies serve as transitional layers between the more public site edge and the more private building envelope, adding further protection. Foundation shrubs accentuate, soften, and protect the building edge. When shrubs (naturalness) are well tended (caring cues) and do not block window views (human scale), they are highly desired by older adults and family members. The intent is to provide a layer of implied protection rather than to impose a barrier, which suggests that older adults are cut off from the world or put away for life. Ivy or other vegetation on exterior walls offers another level of protection, while pitched roofs visible from the ground assure people that the building edge is intact. Although the assisted living building in figure 5.9 was disliked by older adults because of its age (to be discussed later in the chapter), the wrought iron fence and foundation shrubs are features of enclosure that were rated favorably by older adults and family members. The front lawn, steps, and portico are also transitional layers.

53

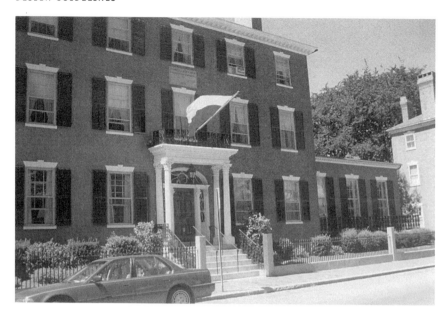

Figure 5.9. *The wrought iron fence and foundation shrubs provide layers of enclosure, while the front lawn and portico offer transitional layers between the public site edge and the private building. Older buildings were favored by family members but were associated with potential maintenance and accessibility problems by older adults.*

Partially Enclose Balconies. Private unit balconies can provide a sense of personal enclosure. Balconies that are recessed and partially enclosed by the building, as opposed to cantilevered balconies, imply protection. This is particularly evident in figure 5.10. The balcony over the entry portico was considered unsafe, while the adjacent, recessed, upper-story balcony was more favorably viewed from a security standpoint. In fact, some family members feared that vulnerable older persons might fall from the balcony over the entry. That does not mean that balconies must be inset into the building. In fact, balconies can be partially enclosed by walls that project beyond the façade, as shown in figure 5.11. Regardless of how balconies are enclosed, it is important to make sure that they are deep enough to accommodate outdoor furniture, activities such as gardening and socializing, and wheelchairs.

Consider Bay and Bow Windows. Bay windows with 30-degree and 45-degree angles, square bay windows, and bow windows also provide a sense of personal enclosure. They project beyond the façade and, compared to conventional windows, provide more light from multiple directions and an enhanced view of the surrounding landscape. Figure 5.11 depicts three bay windows aligned one on top of the other from the building foundation to the roof overhang, while figure 5.12 shows bay windows that are clearly raised above ground level. The alignment of the bay windows in figure 5.11 reduces the perceived projection of the window and may provide a more secure feeling as a result. The research that serves as a basis for this book did not confirm desirable variations of bay windows because of limited depictions of these features in the assisted living environments that were studied. Nevertheless, it is hypothesized that bay windows in various combinations may be relevant design features.

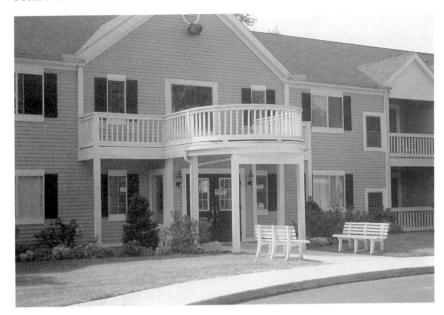

Figure 5.10. *Consumers perceived balconies that are recessed and partially enclosed as safer than balconies that project beyond the façade. Wood siding is a natural material that consumers viewed favorably.*

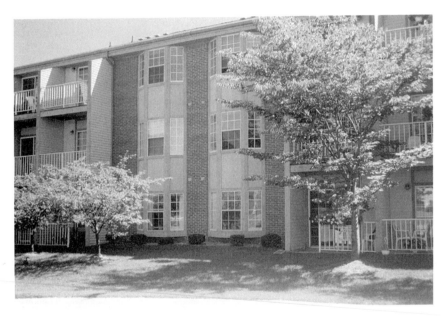

Figure 5.11. *Balconies can also be partially enclosed by walls that project beyond the façade. Bay windows are elements of personal enclosure. When they are aligned from the building foundation to the roofline, they may provide a greater feeling of protection.*

Use Roof Articulations Cautiously. Several theorists have asserted that the roof should be experienced from the outside and the inside to provide people with a basic sense of shelter (Alexander et al., 1977; Jacobson et al., 2002). A pitched roof with articulations such as dormers and cupolas makes it possible to experience the roof from the outside. To be experienced from the inside, the roof must also include living quarters within its volume that reveal the roof shape. Although family members viewed dormers and other roof articulations as familiar housing cues, older adults believed that dormers with windows reflected undesirable and unusable attic space within the building. Where dormers obviously included false windows, as in figure 5.13, the issue of authenticity arose.

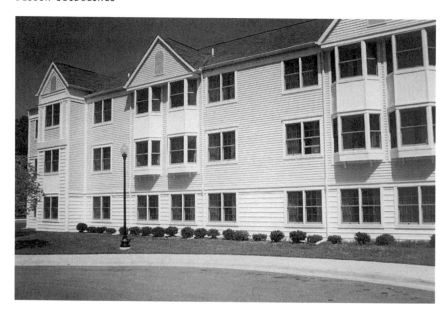

Figure 5.12. *Bay windows above ground level may feel less secure.*

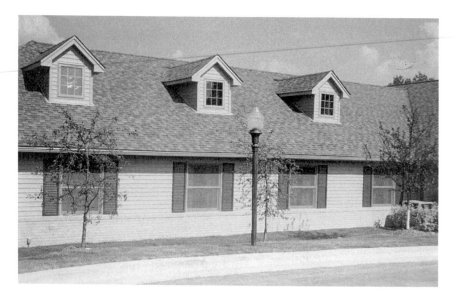

Figure 5.13. *Older adults believed that dormers with windows reflect undesirable and unusable attic space within the building. Dormers with fake windows were considered unauthentic. Changes in material provide the building with a base and help to reduce the massiveness of the façade. Immature trees and sparse vegetation, however, detract from the surrounding landscape.*

Dormers were then considered fake and useless and evoked additional negative reactions among older persons. Thus, roof articulations probably should not be used to imply roof living. Dormers and cupolas that serve another purpose and are useful, as when dormers include air vents rather than windows, are recommended to reconcile differences between family members and older persons (fig. 5.14). Other roof articulations, such as cresting, finials, and weather vanes, are also recommended as familiar housing cues.

Caring Cues

Provide Seating That Encourages Social Interaction. Seating at the entry was a welcoming feature for both older adults and family members. It provides consumers with a place to rest, observe from a point of security, wait for a ride, visit, and socialize. When chairs were stacked up or

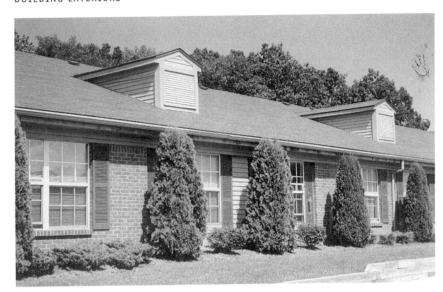

Figure 5.14. *Older adults considered dormers with air vents more useful and acceptable. Both groups of consumers favored lush landscaping provided by foundation shrubs and mature trees.*

arranged haphazardly, however, both older adults and family members viewed seating negatively. Such arrangements suggested that older adults had been "put out to pasture" with no other place to go. In contrast, chairs that are arranged in small groupings, face to face, at right angles, or side by side enhance interaction. Usability is important, too. Outdoor chairs with arm rests on both sides make it easier for older adults to sit down and stand up. Chairs in entries that are protected from the sun are also more comfortable.

Consider Various Combinations of Glazing at the Front Entry. Other front entry features were inviting to consumers. The door itself, when painted a color that contrasts with the exterior of the building, marks the entry and beckons people to approach. Glazed doors, semicircular or elliptical fanlights with sidelights, and rectangular transom windows and sidelights provide glimpses of what is inside the building and can alleviate fears of the unknown. A visible interior entry light is also a welcoming feature (fig. 5.15).

Emphasize Signs of Human Occupancy. Both older adults and family members favorably evaluated assisted living environments with features that imply human presence and nearby support. For example, flat and walkable sidewalks that encircle the site or link the driveway to the entry are welcoming for people. A combination of open and drawn window curtains as well as open and closed windows provides variation and suggests that people are inside the building. The presence of seating and picnic tables, as shown in figure 5.6, is also a sign of human occupancy, even when they are located in front of the building. Detailing such as the window muntins, lintels, and quoins in the building shown in figure 5.8 implies careful attention to the act of building and provides human scale, as discussed later in the chapter.

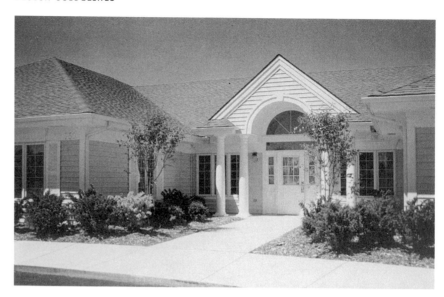

Figure 5.15. *Glazing at the front door is a welcoming feature and helps to prepare consumers for what is inside the building.*

Maintain the Building and Landscaping Reasonably Rather than with Perfection. Care can be exhibited through maintenance. Findings from the studies suggest that the degree of maintenance is important. For instance, participants in the studies verbally indicated that "neatness," "cleanliness," and "freshness" are important. Well-tended shrubs and freshly painted porch railings are examples. That is not to say that everything should be spotless, sterile, or perfect. In fact, participants noted that one of the window shutters in figure 5.16 needed repair, and this slight imperfection was familiar. If lawns were brown and needed watering, however, or bushes were overgrown, these imperfections seemed to be considered more significant and evoked negative reactions. Family members also linked poor maintenance with cheap or low-cost environments.

Consider Older Buildings for Adaptive Reuse on a Case-by-Case Basis. The issue of maintenance was also influenced by the age of buildings. Family members believed that older persons would be able to identify with older buildings and rated such environments favorably as familiar housing (see fig. 5.9). This is consistent with research indicating that the general public prefers buildings and places that look historical (Nasar, 1997). Older adults, however, associated older buildings, including those that had been updated and were in good condition, with potential maintenance problems and rated these environments much less favorably. They also believed older buildings would have outdated heating and cooling systems and would present accessibility problems that affect usability. They rated new construction much more favorably. Previous research indicates that older buildings are usually preferred over modern ones when building maintenance is controlled (Herzog and Gale, 1996; Herzog and Shier, 2000). Thus, the expensive remodeling of older buildings to incorporate an assisted living environment should be

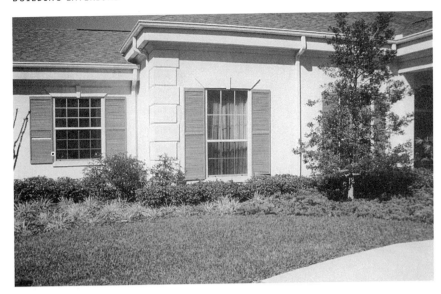

Figure 5.16. Small imperfections, such as a window shutter in need of minor repair, are a familiar cue.

considered cautiously on a case-by-case basis, depending on the marketing realities of individual communities.

Select Light Colors for Façades. Building colors seem to be associated with care as well. Nassauer (1995) asserted that, in the Midwest, white-painted buildings and fences are indicative of care. She did not offer an explanation of why white is more indicative of care than are other colors, but findings from the studies for this book suggest that white or light colors in general are considered fresh and clean. Light colors are also cheerful and bright, which makes it easier for older adults to see. Painting other features, such as window shutters and front doors, a color that contrasts with the façade is desirable for emphasis.

Human Scale

When Economies of Scale Permit, Limit Buildings to One Story. Older adults stressed the need for one-story, low buildings. This desire can be partly attributed to the usability of the environment. Older adults viewed one-story structures as more convenient and accessible, especially if they might need to be evacuated in an emergency. They commented that they would not have to rely on stairs or elevators. The desirability of one-story buildings can also be attributed to human scale. Many older adults revealed that a two-story building height contributed to perceptions of massiveness, while one-story buildings provided a "bungalow feel." The need for one-story buildings to enhance usability and human scale was less important to family members. Nevertheless, when economies of scale permit, it is advisable to build one-story structures for older adults.

Consider One-Story Entries. In a similar vein, the height of entries can greatly affect human scale. As discussed previously, entries such as porte-cocheres were disliked as unfamiliar housing cues. They were also disliked when they were large in relation to the rest of the building and were considered intrusive, heavy, and overbearing (see fig. 5.1). Porticos and porches were more familiar housing cues that were rated favorably by older adults and family members. Human scale, however, also affected the desirability of these familiar entries. For example, a porch was rated positively when it was one story (fig. 5.6) but was considered ostentatious and oversized when it was a two-story, full-façade entry (fig. 5.17). Thus, one-story entries are recommended.

Reduce the Perceived Massing of Façades. Many strategies can be used to reduce the perceived massing of the building façade. For example, cross gables (fig. 5.18), a variety of rooflines (fig. 5.8), a combination of building materials side by side (fig. 5.8), and a change in materials that provides the building with a base (fig. 5.13) help to reduce the long, blank nature of assisted living façades and to create a human scale. Different-sized gables positioned at varying distances, building setbacks, and window and balcony shapes can add depth to the façade and enhance human scale as well.

Accentuate Smaller Parts of the Building. Attention to smaller parts of the building as opposed to elements that are large in relation to the body helps to create a feeling of diminutiveness. These include small foundation shrubs, low fencing, outdoor lamps or lampposts, and building materials such as thin wood siding, brickwork, and tile roofs. Detailing such as spandrels and balustrades around porches and balconies, window trim, lintels or arches, keystones, louvered or paneled shutters, string courses or quoins, bargeboard, and cornices at eave lines enhance the human scale of façades. Color contrast can be used to emphasize ornamentation. Features such as thin, one-story columns, fluted pilasters, entablatures, potted plants, fanlights, and sidelights also en-

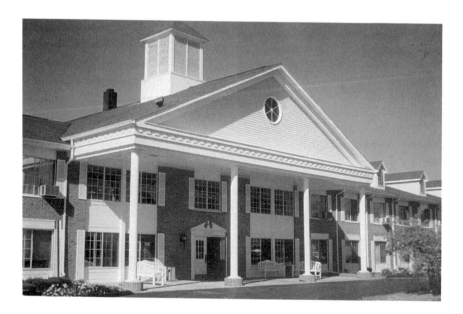

Figure 5.17. *A two-story, full-façade entry often appears massive and oversized.*

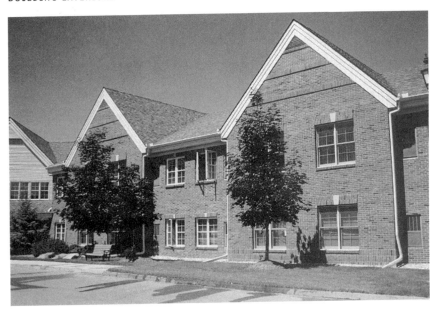

Figure 5.18. *Cross gables help to reduce the perceived massiveness of this building.*

hance human scale at the entry. The assisted living building in figure 5.8 has a human scale because of the combination of building materials, quoins, lintels, small foundation shrubs, and varying rooflines. Consumers considered buildings that did not accentuate smaller parts bare and institutional.

Use Window Dimensions That Relate to the Human Body. While both older adults and family members indicated that they preferred large windows or even double windows to maximize views and natural light, they also expressed a preference for muntins that separate glass panes into smaller units. This may fracture views, but it also enhances the feeling of enclosure and human scale. In addition, consumers stressed that it is important for windows to be low enough for seated people to see out but high enough off the ground to assure protection. Tall, vertical windows were preferred over shorter, wide windows. This is consistent with Boudon's analysis of modernist houses built by Le Corbusier in France. Boudon found that a succession of occupants had replaced wide windows with narrow, small-paned windows in most of the houses (cited in Jacobson et al., 2002).

Naturalness

Use Natural Building Materials Contextually. Building materials can be considered modified elements of nature when used authentically. Both older adults and family members in the Northeast and Midwest rated assisted living buildings that included wood siding (see fig. 5.10) or wood in combination with brick (see fig. 5.8) very favorably. Tile roofs were also rated favorably, even though they are not indigenous to the Midwest or Northeast. In contrast, synthetic materials such as stucco were viewed negatively. This is consistent with previous research indicating that natural building materials, such as fieldstone and wood, as opposed to synthetic materials or those that appear manufactured en-

61

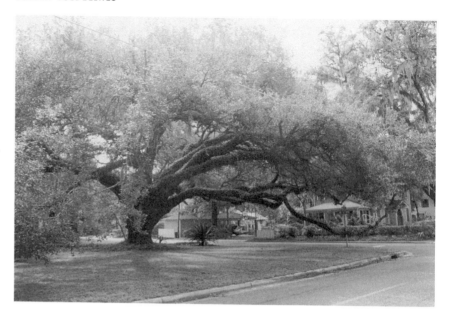

Figure 5.19. *Mature trees provide a layer of enclosure at the site edge, provide protection with sprawling, canopied branches, and enhance views.*

hance preference largely because they serve as connections to the natural environment (Frewald, 1989). Since these building materials have not been studied in the context of all regions throughout the United States, wood and brick are recommended where contextually appropriate. Additional research is needed to determine whether stucco, which is native to certain regions of the country, such as the Southeast and Southwest, is universally less desirable.

Preserve Mature Trees. Trees in general communicate naturalness. Mature trees, however, provide a layer of enclosure at the site edge, provide protection in an umbrella-like way with sprawling, canopied branches, and enhance views (fig. 5.19). Both older adults and family members expressed a strong desire for mature trees as opposed to newer, "stick" trees. Unlike older buildings, which were associated with potential maintenance problems, older trees were not associated with maintenance, such as pruning branches or raking leaves. Thus, it is advisable to preserve older trees with new construction, locating and configuring the building around existing trees on the site.

Add Lush Landscaping. Landscaping enriches and softens the building and offers stimulating views. Landscape elements such as small lawns and foundation shrubs, as shown in figure 5.14, are direct connections to the outdoors and were noted favorably by consumers. These elements should be well tended, should not obstruct views from windows, and should be of a human scale. In contrast, the immature trees and sparse vegetation of figure 5.13 led consumers to rate this environment less favorably even though it includes many of the same architectural features of the assisted living building in figure 5.14. Flowers and other potted plants at the entry were also desirable. Pots bring flowers closer to eye level and provide stimulating colors and fragrances.

CHAPTER 6

Interior Entries

First impressions are more than just a curbside view of the overall building and surrounding landscape. Equally important is the first impression that older adults and family members receive when they pass through the front door of an assisted living building. The interior entry is intended to be welcoming both visually and as a place to use physically. If it is a pleasing space, consumers are more likely to venture onward. The interior entry, as the main artery of the building, then guides occupants to adjacent spaces, such as a common living room or common dining room. The interior entry is also intended to be a transitional space. It offers people who are entering the building the opportunity to orient themselves. Similarly, it offers consumers who are leaving a chance to adjust from one experience inside to another in the outside community.

The following research-based design guidelines contain many ideas for creating an entry that will make an assisted living building just as welcoming inside as it is outside. The guidelines also address features that support patterns of use for both older adults and family members. Design attributes that should be avoided based on consumer input are identified. As with the previous chapter on building exteriors, the guidelines on interior entries are supplemented with photographs and are organized according to the conceptual framework that emerged from the research that serves as the basis for this book.

Familiar Housing Cues

Avoid the Built-in Information Desk and Consider a Movable Piece of Furniture. Like the porte-cochere on the outside of an assisted living building, the information desk with a built-in counter in the interior entry was considered by family members to be oversized and unfamiliar. For example, the information desk beside the front doors in figure 6.1 was considered obtrusive and a barrier between staff and consumers. It was also perceived as a nurses' station and evoked images of hospitals and nursing homes. When a built-in counter was less conspicuous, as in figure 6.2, family members still rated it unfavorably. The counter built into the wall suggested that a concierge or clerk would check visitors into a hotel. A small, movable desk that might be encountered in the foyer, living room, or study of a single-family house, such as the one in figure 6.3, was a more familiar housing cue. Family members also rated interior entries without an information or check-in desk very favorably.

In contrast, the information desk was a much more important feature for older adults. Many believed that a desk was welcoming and suggested that a staff member would be nearby to greet people, ease

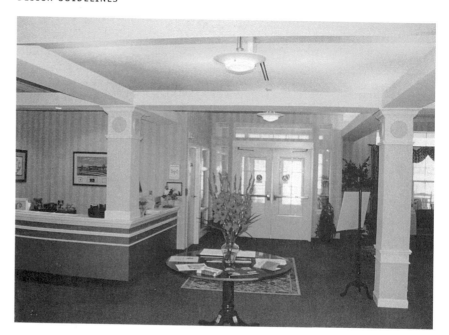

Figure 6.1. *An information desk with a built-in counter is often oversized and an unfamiliar cue. It is also perceived as a barrier between staff and consumers.*

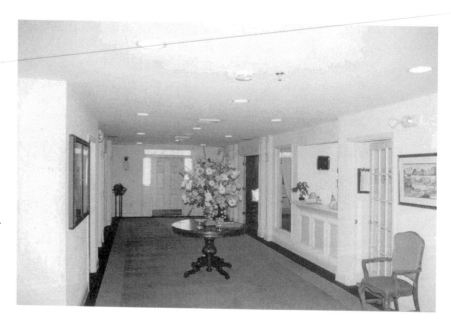

Figure 6.2. *An information desk with a smaller built-in counter is less conspicuous but is still an unfamiliar housing cue for family members. Older adults stressed the need for an information desk and viewed smaller ones more favorably even when they were unfamiliar housing cues.*

apprehensions, engage in conversation, answer questions, and offer assistance, which communicate caring. Even when an information desk resembled something you would typically encounter in a hotel lobby, as in figure 6.2, older adults still rated this feature favorably. When the desk was too large and obtrusive, however, as in figure 6.1, the need for a familiar housing cue became more important to older adults than was the desire for a friendly information desk.

To reconcile differences between both groups, consider movable pieces of furniture, such as writing tables, secretary desks, consoles, and commodes or bureaus with hinged lids. Large executive desks, such as the one in figure 6.4, should be considered cautiously. For some family

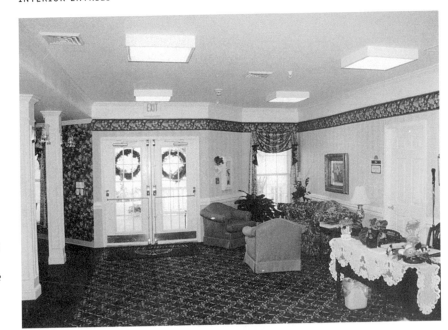

Figure 6.3. *A small, movable desk that might be encountered in the foyer, living room, or study of a single-family house is a more familiar housing cue. When the path from the front door into the entry is clear, it is easier for older adults to navigate the space.*

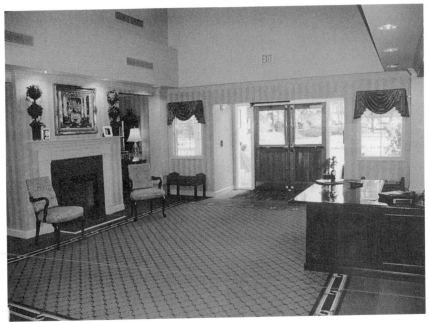

Figure 6.4. *Large executive desks can resemble workstations and are less desirable. Familiar housing cues such as a fireplace, artwork above the fireplace, window treatments, and table lamps are favorable features. Older adults responded positively to interior entries that are well defined with walls. Visual access to other spaces was important to family members and is provided by the wall openings on each side of the fireplace. Older adults also responded positively to entries with clear passageways from the front door, doors with glazing and windows that provide views to the outside, and carpeting that reduces glare.*

members, they resembled workstations and were too business-like and overpowering. The use of smaller desks, a feature of human scale, may necessitate proximity to a workroom or office with storage that is shared with administration and other staff.

Reference Interior Features of the Single-Family House. In addition to movable desks, other features that evoked images of the single-family house were rated favorably. In particular, the fireplace was a desirable symbol in the interior entry of assisted living buildings, even though it was associated with the entry or foyer of larger homes (fig. 6.4). Family

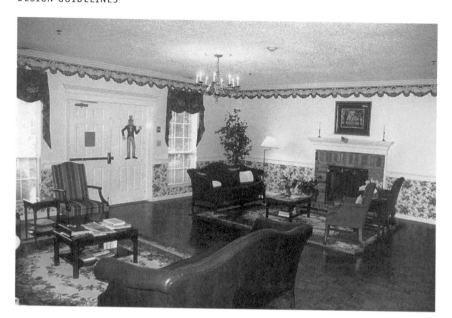

Figure 6.5. The chandelier is a familiar housing cue in the interior entry. Holiday decorations, such as the one located on the front door of this entry, are sometimes perceived as childlike and inappropriate.

members placed a greater emphasis than did older adults on residential décor, but both groups appreciated the selective use of artwork above the fireplace or elsewhere on walls, window treatments, and lamps on tables, as shown in figure 6.4. Not surprisingly, bare walls were less desirable. Family members also identified ornate chandeliers as a positive feature, as depicted in the assisted living building entry in figure 6.5.

Features that are used in an unfamiliar way should be avoided. Older adults responded negatively to certain holiday decorations, such as the cardboard image of Uncle Sam taped to the front door in figure 6.5. They believed that such decorations were childlike rather than festive and were inappropriate with formal furnishings. Family members did not find the decorations problematic and even thought they were endearing. The interior entry shown in figure 6.6 was intended to bring the outdoors inside. Green carpeting, pots and planters, wallpaper that simulates brick, and wrought iron furniture in the interior entry was disconcerting to both older adults and family members and did not meet their expectations for how an interior space should look.

Protective Enclosure

Create a Well-Defined Space. An interior entry in an assisted living building may simply consist of a few floor tiles. In this scenario, the front door usually opens directly into a space such as a living room. The interior entry may also be an open space that visually and spatially links other rooms to add interest and allow occupants to preview rooms before entering them. The entry may also be a room with clearly defined edges and minimal openings between adjacent spaces.

Older adults put a greater emphasis on interior entries with well-defined edges. The interior entry in figure 6.4, for example, was rated favorably. The wallcovering that creates a horizontal band around the room, the carpet pattern, and the ceiling soffit accentuate the edges. Visual access to the adjacent living room is provided through door open-

66

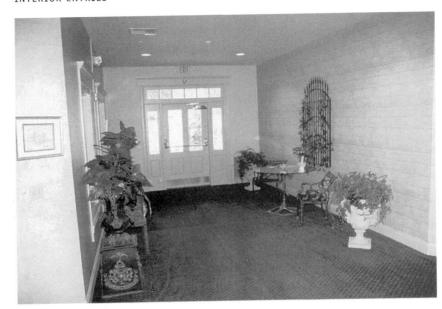

Figure 6.6. *Although this interior entry was intended to bring the outdoors inside, the space does not meet consumers' expectations about the appearance and intended use of an interior entry in an assisted living building.*

ings on each side of the fireplace. The interior entry in figure 6.7 is clearly a separate room and does not provide visual access to spaces other than what is in front of the occupant. Older adults, however, rated this assisted living entry and others like it favorably as well. This is inconsistent with empirical studies of exterior built space, which indicate that people prefer defined openness (Nasar, 1999). In contrast, family members perceived more enclosed entries, such as the ones shown in figures 6.2, 6.6, and 6.7, unfavorably as long hallways. To meet the needs of both consumer groups, designers should perhaps explore ways to define entry spaces reasonably well for older adults and also provide some visual access to other spaces for family members. Changes in floor material, half-walls, and furniture arrangements that separate spaces do not seem to be sufficient to define the extent of an interior entry.

Caring Cues

Provide a Small Seating Area. As with exterior entries such as porches, seating in interior entries is a welcoming feature for both older adults and family members. It provides consumers with a place to rest, wait for a ride or visitor, converse with a staff member behind a desk, or watch people entering and exiting the building. Seating consisting of two or three armchairs or upholstered chairs clustered together along the edge of the room is desirable. Larger seating areas consisting of couches typically found in a living room were less desirable in the entry. Interior entries that did not provide seating at all were unfavorably rated.

Emphasize Color. Many interior entries that integrated bright colors were well received by consumers. Colorful flower arrangements, for instance, caught the attention of both older adults and family members. Older adults were also drawn to carpeting that included bright colors. For example, carpeting with a bold red center and green border was favorably noted in many instances and provided a contrast against more

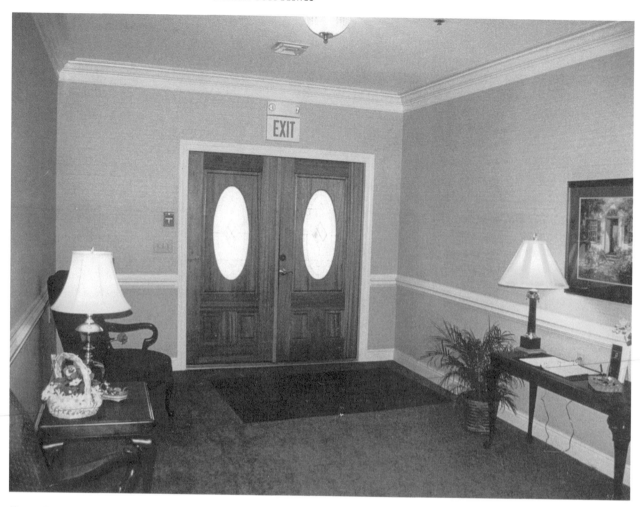

Figure 6.7. *This entry is a separate room and does not provide visual access to other spaces. Older adults viewed enclosed entries favorably, while family members perceived them as long hallways.*

neutral wall colors such as yellow and beige. Even purple carpeting was favorably rated. For many older adults, the bright colors were cheerful and uplifting, provided positive stimulation, and animated the environment. Colors of medium tone may also help to compensate for changes in color perception that accompany old age. In contrast, older adults found dark floor colors such as brown and green, which are common in assisted living entries to facilitate maintenance, dreary and bland. Dark colors also diminished the ability of older adults to see effectively in the environment.

Human Scale

Explore Ceiling Variations. A change in ceiling height is often used to create a memorable experience of arrival. In many houses designed by Frank Lloyd Wright (1954), visitors are led through a front door into an intimate space with a low ceiling to enhance human scale. When visitors move through the compressed entry into a living room, typically with a height of one and one-half or two stories, there is an explosion of space. The living room often seems larger because of the compression that visitors experience before entering the room. In assisted living buildings, the reverse is often true. Consumers pass through two-story

68

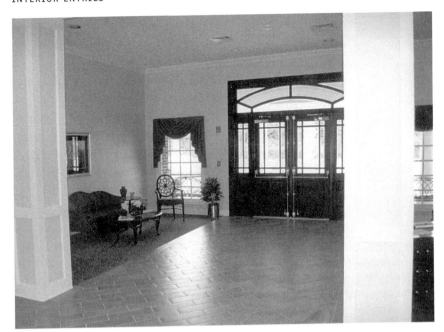

Figure 6.8. *The one-and-one-half-story entry appears massive to consumers. The reflected glare from the floor tile diminishes usability and drew negative reactions from older adults.*

entries into one-story common living rooms. The two-story entry may be the highest space of a surrounding one-story building or may visually connect the ground floor with a second floor.

Older adults rated two-story interior entryways unfavorably. Even the one-and-one-half-story entry in the assisted living building in figure 6.8 appeared immense to older adults because of the volume of space. This is reinforced by the size of the front doors and the thick columns. Older persons stressed the need for entries with lower ceilings. This is not surprising; they also articulated a desire for one-story, low buildings. The ceiling height of interior entryways was not salient in family members' perceptions. Thus, a lower ceiling height is recommended.

Spatial diversity is possible even without a two-story or one-and-one-half-story space. The low tray ceiling of the assisted living interior entry in figure 6.9 and the low barrel-vaulted ceiling in figure 6.10 were well received by both groups of consumers. When cove lighting was integrated into the ceiling treatments to provide indirect lighting, older adults rated the entries in figures 6.9 and 6.10 even more favorably because of enhanced usability of the space. It is important to explore ways in which ceiling shapes (cathedral, tray, vault, dome, dropped) and treatments can add drama to the space and enhance human scale and usability at the same time. Because of physical and sensory changes that affect mobility, it is less feasible to provide spatial diversity at the floor plane through changes in level.

Accentuate Decorative Moldings. Attention to smaller parts of the interior entry as opposed to elements that are large in relation to the body helps to create a feeling of diminutiveness. Moldings in varying sizes, shapes, and combinations can add decorative interest and enhance human scale. The ceiling can be articulated with a cornice molding, the

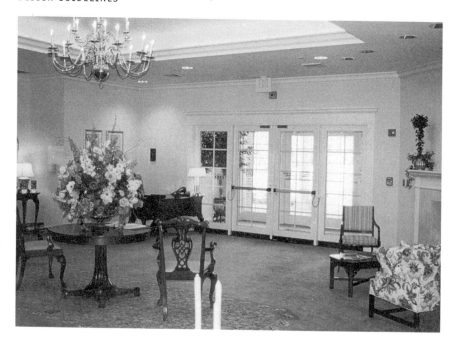

Figure 6.9. *The low tray ceiling with cove lighting adds spatial diversity while enhancing human scale and usability. The use of moldings throughout also adds to the human scale of the space. The doors with glazing and sidelights provide views to the outdoors, and the flowers on the center table are direct connections to nature.*

floor can be offset with a baseboard, and the wall can be divided with applied molding to create a variety of patterns. Moldings can also be used to articulate ceiling shapes or openings such as doors and windows and to decorate fireplace mantels, columns, and pilasters. Human scale is enhanced in the interior entryway of figure 6.9, where moldings are used in a variety of ways.

Usability

Keep Passageways Clear. As the main artery of the building, the interior entry is a passageway and link to other spaces. Accessibility along the main artery is an important concern for older adults. As discussed in chapter 1, 59 percent of assisted living residents are ambulatory, but 41 percent require the assistance of a mobility aid such as a wheelchair, walker, or cane (Assisted Living Federation of America [ALFA], 2000). Assistive devices often necessitate attention to the amount of floor area, the width of spaces, and the distance between furniture. Older adults indicated that it was very important to provide interior entries that are roomy and uncluttered without sacrificing human scale. In particular, an entry with a path from the front door that is clear and easy to navigate was favorably received. Figures 6.3 and 6.4 are examples. Other assisted living entries that provided enough room to navigate around a central focal point, such as a table with a flower arrangement, were also well received (see fig. 6.10). In addition, a clear central path provides a comfortable distance between consumers who may be sitting in the entry and those passing through. Although a clear path was not salient in family members' perceptions, it is still important to consider accessibility for older consumers.

Avoid Glare. Family members favorably rated genuine wood flooring and Pergo laminate flooring as natural finish materials. In contrast, older

70

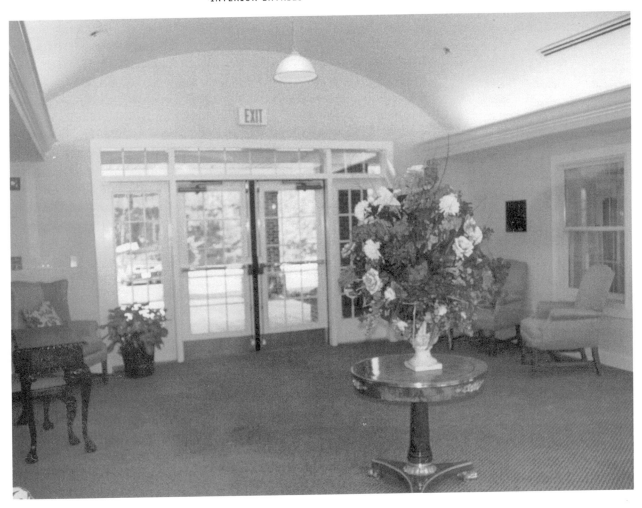

Figure 6.10. *This low barrel-vaulted ceiling also integrates cove lighting. Sufficient floor area allows consumers to navigate freely around the center table in the entry. The flowers on the table also create a colorful focal point.*

adults rated wood floors unfavorably because of reflected glare from entry windows and door glazing. Tile floors were rated unfavorably for the same reason (see fig. 6.8). Carpeting was favored among older adults as a floor covering to minimize glare in the entry. Family members also favored the use of area rugs over hardwood floors as a familiar housing cue and as a way to break up the entry space. Older adults, however, considered area rugs over hardwood or tile floors tripping hazards unless rugs were inset to provide a level surface, as shown in figure 6.8. To reconcile differences between both groups, use matte finishes for flooring, make sure that all floor materials are level, and investigate devices for sun control on the outside and the inside of the building that are familiar housing cues.

Naturalness

Enhance Views to the Outdoors. It is advantageous to provide consumers with glimpses of what is inside an assisted living building when they are approaching from the street or drive. Glazed doors and fanlights or transom windows with sidelights at the exterior entry can be welcoming and alleviate fears of the unknown. In a similar manner, glazing that provides views from the interior entry to the outdoors is desirable

71

to older adults and family members. Views to the outside allow consumers to prepare for the transition between the inside and outside of the building as they exit. Views to the outside also help to keep older adults, who spend most of their time indoors, connected to landscaping, wildlife, the seasons, and the time of day. In addition, views to outdoor activities are other sources of stimulation. In the interior entry of the assisted living building shown in figure 6.9, the double front doors and sidelights are fully glazed to maximize views to the outside even when occupants are seated. Older adults and family members rated such entries favorably as a result. The doors, sidelights, and adjacent windows in the interior entry of figure 6.4 were also well received, and the carpeting helped to reduce glare. In contrast, solid doors and doors with frosted glass were viewed unfavorably even when windows were provided in the entry near the front doors.

Create a Focal Point with Fresh Flowers. Live flowers are natural elements that provide stimulating colors and fragrances. Flower arrangements in vases or pots can also provide a focal point for the interior entry. The arrangements on the center tables in the interior entries in figures 6.9 and 6.10 drew strong positive reactions from older adults and family members. Even though the tables blocked the path from the front door, older adults believed there was sufficient room to navigate around the center tables. Flower arrangements can also be positioned on small tables at the edges of entries, on fireplace mantles, and on information desks.

CHAPTER 7

Common Living Rooms

The living room of an assisted living building is usually a separate space that can be entered directly from the interior entry. Sometimes it can be immediately accessed from the front door and doubles as an entrance. As a semipublic space, the living room is intended to be used by residents, family members, staff, and other visitors for socialization and a variety of individual and group activities. The design and décor of the living room also project an image that creates an atmosphere. The image is intended to attract prospective consumers and to appeal to current residents and their family members.

The following research-based design guidelines focus on the visual aspects of living rooms in assisted living buildings as well as physical features that affect the abilities of consumers to function effectively in the space. The guidelines are supplemented with photographs that were used during data collection and are organized according to the conceptual framework presented in chapter 4.

Familiar Housing Cues

Provide a Less Formal Décor. Furniture style and arrangement, lighting, artwork, and accessories, as well as the color, texture, and pattern of upholstery, window treatments, wallpapers, paint finishes, and floor coverings, are elements of décor that contribute to the living room atmosphere. Sometimes the living room in an assisted living building is envisioned as a formal and elegant showplace with well-coordinated fabrics and finishes to present a marketing image for prospective consumers. In other instances, the living room may be more casual and present a lived-in look that suggests the room is used on a daily basis.

Family members rated living rooms with a less formal décor desirably. In particular, the living room in the assisted living building in figure 7.1 was noted by many as a cozy space that resembled a den or family room they would encounter in a single-family house. The painting over the fireplace, pillows on the couch, and upholstered furniture were favorable features. In contrast, more formal arrangements such as the living room in figure 7.2 evoked images of a funeral parlor, were considered cold and stiff, and were rated unfavorably. This may be because the informal family room as well as the home office and study have replaced the formal living room in newer single-family houses. Older adults placed much less emphasis on the formality of the décor in the living room. Although they also rated the living room in figure 7.2 unfavorably, features such as dark wall colors and uncomfortable furniture that affect usability influenced their perceptions instead. Similarly, the pillows and overstuffed furniture in the living room in figure

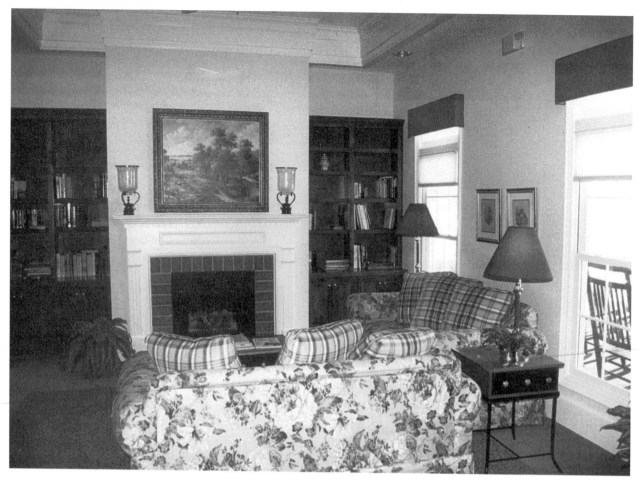

Figure 7.1. *Family members favored living rooms with a cozy, less formal décor. Wood bookshelves, the artwork above the fireplace, window treatments, and table lamps are familiar housing cues. The furniture in the room is grouped around two focal points—a fireplace and bookshelves—that work together. The furniture is grouped too closely together for older adults, however, making the room appear crowded and difficult to navigate. The overstuffed couch with loose pillows for back support also drew negative responses from older adults. Features such as divided lights in windows, the fireplace mantel, and smaller bookcases enhance human scale.*

7.1 make it difficult for older adults to rise from a seated position, affecting usability. These features will be described in more detail later in the chapter. To meet the needs of family members, a less formal décor in the living room of assisted living buildings is recommended.

Reference Living Room Features of the Single-Family House. Features that referenced the living room of the single-family house were rated favorably and are suggested. Both older adults and family members considered the fireplace a desirable element in the living room of assisted living buildings. Even with the advancement of heating technology, the fireplace, including the hearth, surround, and mantel, remains a strong symbol of domesticity in the United States. Wood shelves, which add naturalness, were also familiar living room cues and were rated favorably. The shelves can be used for books, as in figure 7.1, or to display ornaments as well as books, as in figure 7.3. Family members placed a greater emphasis on residential décor than did older adults, but both groups appreciated the selective use of artwork above the fireplace or elsewhere on walls, window treatments, and lamps on tables, as shown in figure 7.1. Not surprisingly, bare living room walls, as shown in figure 7.4, were less desirable and were considered stark and impersonal by both groups of consumers.

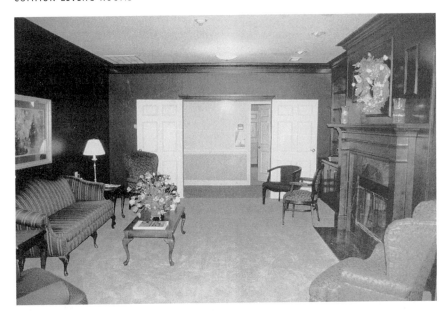

Figure 7.2. More formal living room arrangements evoke images of funeral parlors. The dark wall colors, dark and uncomfortable furniture, and lack of natural light also drew negative reactions from older adults.

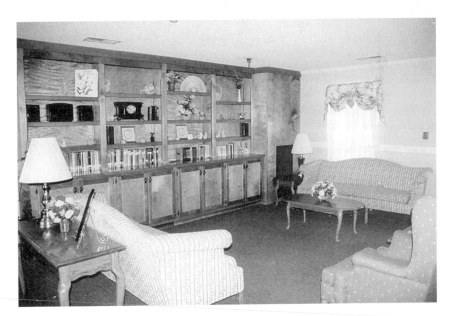

Figure 7.3. Shelves used for ornaments or knickknacks as well as books are familiar housing cues. When the scale of the shelves or wall unit is too large, however, human scale is sacrificed.

Protective Enclosure

Explore Various Ways to Define the Living Space. In the previous chapter, it was noted that older adults favorably rated interior entries that were separate rooms with well-defined edges. Family members desired entries that were less enclosed and provided visual access to other rooms. Some of the living rooms that were included in the research that serves as a basis for this book were separate rooms accessed by separate circulation routes. Other living rooms included circulation routes along the edges of the living room, which provided occupants with the opportunity to view the space without interrupting the activities within. In such instances, the outer walls of the circulation route defined the living room (fig. 7.5). How the room was spatially defined was not salient in consumers' perceptions. Either separate living rooms or living rooms

75

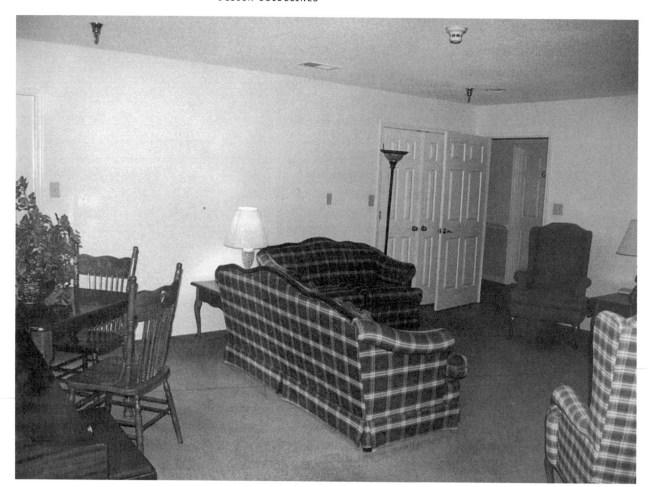

Figure 7.4. *Consumers considered bare walls stark and impersonal.*

Figure 7.5. *The outer walls of a circulation route define this living room. Circulation along the perimeter of the room allows consumers to preview the space without interrupting activities within. Two separate activity areas make it possible for consumers to pursue multiple activities simultaneously. Furniture in the larger activity area is successfully arranged around three focal points—a fireplace, shelves for ornaments, and a television—that work together. In addition, the colorful upholstered chairs and couches stand out against the more neutral wall color and provide padded but firm seating.*

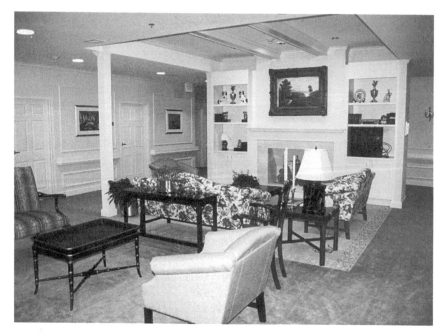

that integrated circulation were desirable if familiar housing cues, human scale, and usability were taken into account. This suggests that designers should continue to explore various ways in which to define the living space.

Caring Cues

Arrange Furniture around a Focal Point. A focal point attracts attention, provides a center of interest, and helps to establish a sense of order in a room. It can be an architectural element such as a fireplace or a window with a pleasing view; a piece of furniture such as a piano, a large-screen television, bookshelves, or a desk; or a furnishing such as a portrait painting, sculpture, decorative rug, or flower arrangement. Focal points can also be reinforced. A fireplace, for example, may include a pair of matching vases or candlesticks on each side of the mantel and a framed picture or decorative mirror above. A larger room may include more than one focal point. In such cases, the focal points can be arranged to work together or the room may be divided into two or more areas to minimize competition between foci.

Living rooms in assisted living buildings that were rated favorably by older adults and family members had furniture arranged around focal points that are familiar housing cues. The furniture in the living room in figure 7.6, for instance, is grouped around the fireplace as a single focal point. In figure 7.1, furniture is arranged around two focal points—a fireplace and bookshelves—that work together. Furniture is successfully arranged around three focal points—a fireplace, shelves that could hold books or ornaments, and a television—in figure 7.5. In contrast, living rooms without focal points, with competing foci, or with furniture arrangements that blocked focal points were less desirable

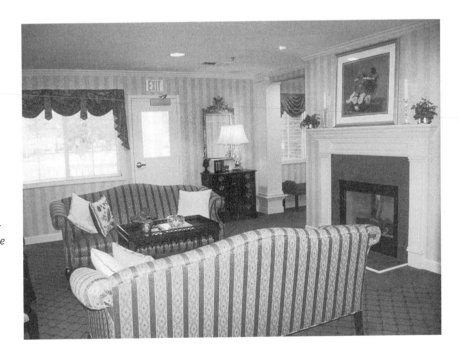

Figure 7.6. Furniture grouped around a single focal point, such as a fireplace, helps to provide order and a center of interest in the room. The colorful carpeting and couches are uplifting and provide contrast against the neutral wall colors. The divided lights in the windows, molding, and fireplace mantel also enhance human scale. In addition, the firm couches make it easier for older adults to rise from a seated position.

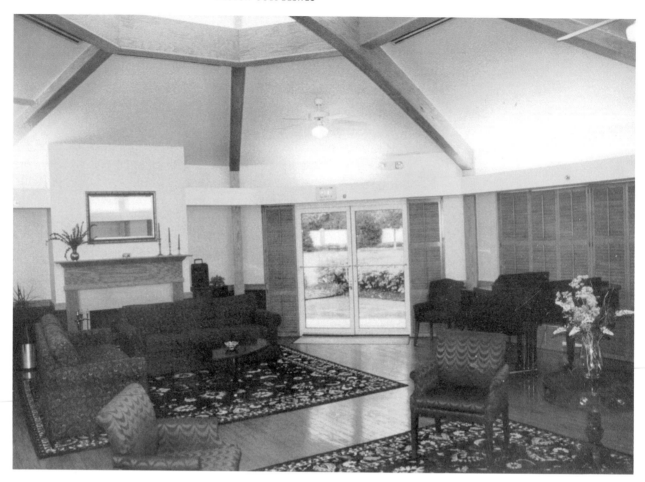

Figure 7.7. *The three focal points—a fireplace, glass doors with a pleasing outdoor view, and piano—in this living room do not work together. As a result, the seating appears scattered and the room is confusing to consumers. The large floor area, distance between the furniture, and ceiling height also contribute to perceptions of massiveness.*

and were confusing to older adults in many cases. The living room in figure 7.7 includes three focal points: a fireplace, glass doors with views to landscaping, and a grand piano. One of the couches, however, blocks the fireplace, both couches are positioned at a great distance from the piano, and some of the chairs are oriented with their backs to the piano. As a result, the focal points compete with one another, and the seating appeared scattered to consumers. Similarly, the living room in figure 7.8 includes a fireplace, a television, and a piano that compete with one another because the furniture is arranged around the perimeter of the room. Several chairs block the television and are oriented with their backs to the television or the fireplace. This suggested to older adults and family members that some occupants would not be able to enjoy these features.

Provide Opportunities for Multiple Activities. Focal points are usually created with certain activities in mind. Older adults and family members appreciated living rooms with focal points that worked together to support a variety of individual and group activities. Activity choices also suggested that older residents would more likely be able to pursue interests that they had developed before moving into an assisted living

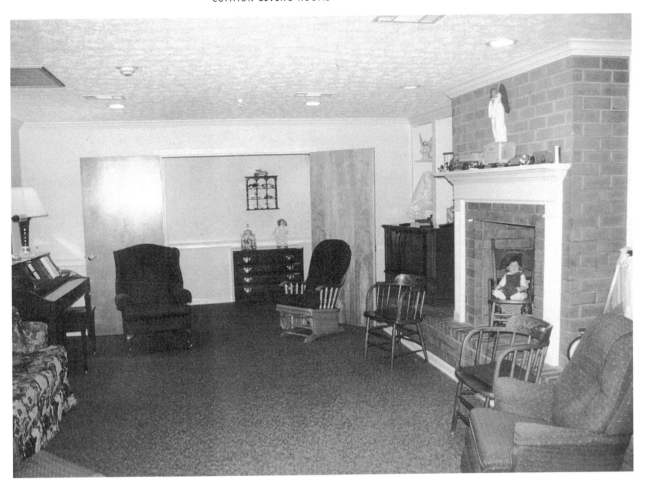

Figure 7.8. *The furniture around the perimeter of this living room blocks several focal points. The room is surrounded by circulation hallways and thus does not provide natural light or views to the outdoors.*

building. Thus, living rooms that provided multiple opportunities for watching television or movies, listening to music, reading, playing board or card games, and conversing were important to consumers. Features that support such activities included armoires or entertainment centers for televisions, pianos, shelves with accessible books, places for reading, small tables for games, and seats arranged at right angles or across from each other at close distances to facilitate private conversations and enhance family visits. Both older adults and family members felt that there should be enough seating to accommodate several occupants.

Consumers viewed separate activity areas in the living room favorably because separate areas suggested that occupants would be able to pursue multiple activities simultaneously in the same room. For example, the living room in figure 7.5 consists of a larger seating area grouped around a fireplace and television and an adjacent smaller seating area. This suggested that some older persons would be able to watch television in the larger area while others were conversing in the smaller area. Similarly, the living room in figure 7.9 includes a game table, a larger seating area for watching television, and a more private, smaller seating area. Although the furniture is positioned too far away for tele-

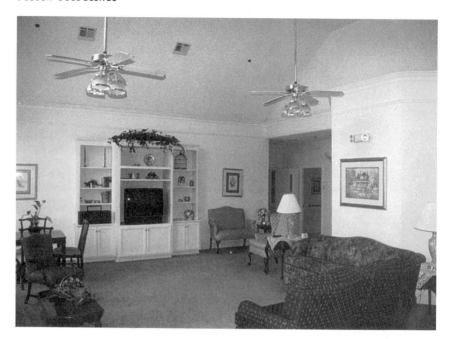

Figure 7.9. *This living room includes multiple activity areas consisting of a game table, a larger seating area for watching television, and a more private seating area for conversation. Plants that are not within reach, such as the one on top of the entertainment center, are difficult for consumers to enjoy.*

vision watching, consumers felt that this living room offered multiple opportunities for activities that could be pursued individually or by different groups of people at the same time. It is important to find the right combination of semiprivate and semipublic areas and to put them together in a way that supports various activities.

Emphasize Cheerful Colors and Avoid Dark Colors. As with interior entries, many of the living rooms that integrated bright colors were considered cheerful and uplifting. They also provided positive stimulation and animated the environment. In particular, older adults and family members were drawn to colorful carpeting and furniture upholstery. The couches and chairs in the living rooms in figures 7.5 and 7.6 stood out against the more neutral wall colors. In contrast, older adults found dark-colored furniture upholstery against dark wall colors problematic (see fig. 7.2). They felt it would be more difficult to find their way in a dark space, affecting usability. They also felt a dark space would be dreary and depressing.

Human Scale

Emphasize Small Spaces. The living room in an assisted living building is sometimes envisioned as a great room, like the ones that are now a central part of newer single-family houses. In such instances, the living room may appear large because of the size of the floor area, the ceiling height, and the way the furniture is arranged. Large living rooms or great rooms in assisted living buildings were not well received by older adults or family members. For example, the large floor area, the distance between the furniture, and the ceiling height and ceiling articulations in figure 7.7 contributed to consumer perceptions of massiveness. When the furniture in the living room was spaced closer together and the floor area was smaller, as in figure 7.10, family members rated such

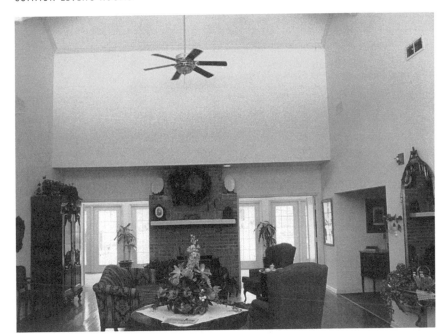

Figure 7.10. *The small floor area and the close spacing of furniture made this living room desirable to family members, but the high ceiling drew negative reactions from older adults. Live plants placed throughout the room are important to all consumers.*

living rooms favorably. They were less concerned about the ceiling height in the room. However, the ceiling height still made the space feel much too large for older adults. This is consistent with the design guidelines in previous chapters. Older adults articulated a desire for a one-story building height and interior entries with lower ceilings. To reconcile differences between both groups of consumers, designers should plan living rooms with smaller floor areas, lower ceilings, and close spacing of furniture. Furniture should not be spaced too closely together, however. The ability to navigate around furniture affects usability and will be discussed later in this chapter. Refer to figure 7.11 for an example of a living room with a human scale that is easy for older persons to navigate.

Focus on Small-Scale Elements. Attention to smaller parts of the living room as opposed to elements that are large in relation to the body helps to create a feeling of diminutiveness. As discussed in chapter 6, moldings of varying sizes, shapes, and combinations can add decorative interest and enhance human scale. Divided lights in windows and ornaments or knickknacks on tables, shelves, and fireplace mantels also enhance human scale (see figs. 7.1 and 7.6). Bookcases are familiar housing cues in living rooms. When they are constructed of wood, they also incorporate naturalness. In addition, smaller bookcases relate to human scale. Multiple, smaller bookcases, as depicted in the living rooms in figures 7.1 and 7.12, were considered more desirable by both older adults and family members than were larger bookcases, like the one shown in figure 7.3.

Provide Room to Navigate around Furniture. The ability to navigate around furniture in living rooms of assisted living buildings is an im-

Usability

81

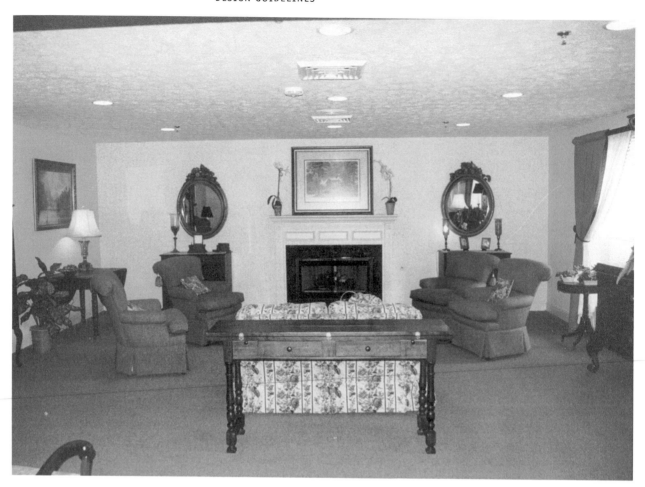

Figure 7.11. *Human scale is evident in this living room with a low ceiling and smaller floor area. The spacing between furniture is close enough for conversation but distant enough to allow older adults to easily navigate the space.*

portant concern for older adults. Difficulty with mobility and the use of assistive devices such as canes and walkers necessitate attention to the amount of floor area and the arrangement of furniture. Roomy and uncluttered living rooms that retained a feeling of human scale were well received by older adults. For example, there is adequate spacing between the chairs and the small sofa in figure 7.11. At the same time, the furniture is close enough together to permit conversation. In contrast, older adults believed that the furniture in figure 7.1 was too close together, making it appear crowded and suggesting that it would be difficult to move throughout the room. Family members, however, favored living rooms with furniture very close together and were less concerned with space around furniture for easy movement. To meet the needs of older adults, arrange furniture to facilitate ambulation throughout the space.

Avoid Overstuffed Furniture. Family members considered overstuffed chairs and couches with large pillows for back support, such as the ones shown in the living room in figure 7.1, comfortable, relaxing, and cozy. Older adults, however, viewed overstuffed seating less favorably. They

82

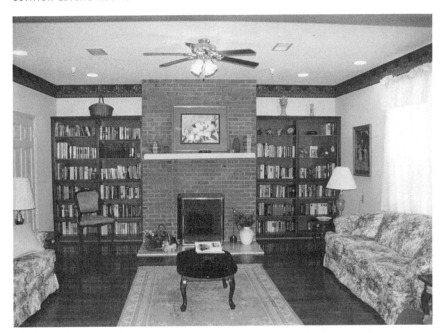

Figure 7.12. *Smaller bookcases are desirable to enhance human scale.*

feared that overstuffed couches and chairs would provide less support and would be difficult to get in and out of as needed. Couches and chairs with padded but firm seating and backs as well as arms were viewed much more favorably by older adults and are recommended (see figs. 7.5, 7.6, and 7.9).

Naturalness

Provide Windows to Enhance Views to the Outdoors. The provision of windows in the living rooms of assisted living buildings to enhance views to the outdoors may seem to be an obvious design suggestion, but several living rooms included in the research that serves as a basis for this book were centrally located spaces, surrounded by hallways or other rooms, and did not include windows or skylights (see figs. 7.2 and 7.8). Both older adults and family members regarded living rooms without windows negatively and indicated that views to the outdoors were needed to maintain connections to nature. The living room in figure 7.1 provides views to the porch outside. Even though the living room in figure 7.7 was disliked because of the scale of the space and the arrangement of the furniture, many consumers commented that the outdoor view was pleasing. In addition to views, windows provide natural light. According to Brawley (1997), research has indicated that people who are deprived of natural light may suffer from sleep disorders, depression, and poor calcium metabolism, which depletes bone mass.

Provide Real Indoor Plants and Flowers. Real plants and flowers are strong connections to nature and provide opportunities for older adults to care for something that is alive. The Eden alternative stresses that continuing contact with plants helps to enliven housing arrangements and provide older adults with a purpose (Thomas, 1996). Both older adults and family members were attracted to flower arrangements and plants positioned on furniture, the floor, or fireplace hearths (see fig. 7.10). Plants that were not within reach, such as the one on top of the entertainment center in figure 7.9, were less desirable. Consumers believed that they could not easily tend such plants and assumed they were artificial.

Chapter 8

Common Dining Rooms

The dining room in an assisted living building is primarily used by older adults for meal consumption. The consumption of food is a necessary activity; eating provides nutrients that sustain life. Meal consumption is also a social activity. Opportunities for interaction with other residents and with staff who care for residents are possible. Socialization may be enhanced during special holiday or birthday celebrations or if family members dine with residents. Sometimes the dining room is also used for other activities such as crafts, games, or entertainment and functions as a multipurpose room. Regardless of the intended activities, the dining room is the most regularly and heavily used common space in an assisted living building. The design and décor of the dining room are also intended to support patterns of use and establish an atmosphere.

The guidelines that follow focus on assisted living dining rooms. Features that are important to consumers as well as attributes that should be avoided are identified. As in the previous chapters that focus on design guidelines, the recommendations in this chapter are supplemented with photographs and are organized according to the conceptual framework that emerged from the research described in the introduction.

Familiar Housing Cues

Provide a More Formal Décor. It was noted in chapter 7 that family members favored living rooms with a less formal décor. Furniture style and arrangement, lighting, artwork, and accessories, as well as the color, texture, and pattern of upholstery, window treatments, wallpapers, paint finishes, and floor coverings, contributed to decorating perceptions. In contrast, family members expressed a desire for a more formal décor in dining rooms, perhaps because the dining room remains one of the most formal rooms in the single-family house today. All of the assisted living dining rooms evaluated in the research were separate spaces and were not part of an open plan that included informal spaces such as kitchens or family rooms.

Features that contributed to perceptions of formality in assisted living dining rooms included brass chandeliers and traditional furniture styles with dark wood, as shown in figure 8.1. Other formal features included linen tablecloths, table settings with napkins and glassware, decorative wallpaper, wainscoting, crown molding, and decorative window treatments (fig. 8.2). Although older adults did not discriminate between assisted living dining rooms with respect to the formality of the

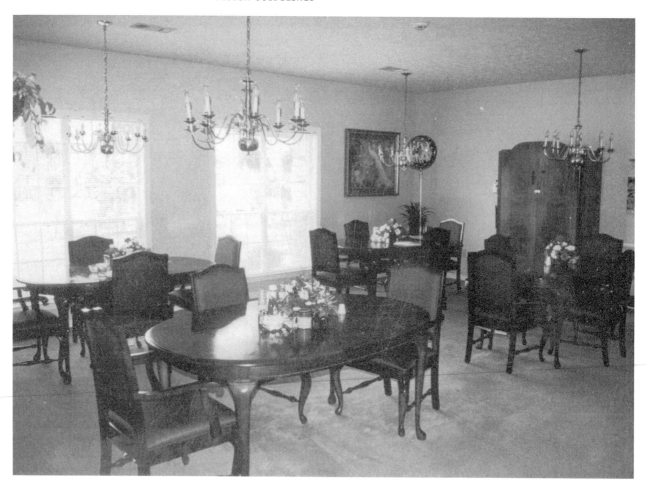

Figure 8.1. *Brass chandeliers and traditional furniture styles with dark wood contribute to perceptions of formality. Family members regarded traditional tables and chairs favorably as familiar housing cues, but older adults found the furniture too dark, which affects usability.*

décor, a more formal arrangement is recommended to meet the needs of family members.

Reference Dining Room Features of the Single-Family House. Many of the features that contributed to a formal décor were also considered by family members to be familiar dining room cues of the single-family house. These included hutches, cabinets, or breakfronts for storing and displaying china and glassware; sideboards, buffets, or servers; chandeliers; window treatments; and artwork on walls. Family members also regarded traditional tables and chairs, such as the ones in figures 8.1 and 8.3, as pieces of furniture you would typically encounter in a single-family house. Older adults placed less emphasis on familiar housing cues and viewed dining rooms more in terms of usability. For example, the darkness of the furniture and the glare off of the polished tabletops in the dining rooms in figures 8.1 and 8.3 suggested that it would be difficult for older adults to function in those spaces. Usability will be discussed in more detail later in the chapter.

Protective Enclosure

Avoid Views from Circulation Routes. In the previous chapter, we saw that the way the living room is spatially defined was not salient in con-

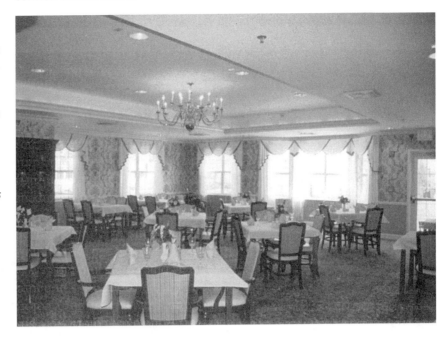

Figure 8.2. *Formal features include linen tablecloths, table settings with linen napkins and glassware, decorative wallpaper, wainscoting, crown molding, and decorative window treatments. Linen tablecloths and napkins and glassware as opposed to plastic or disposable tableware communicate care. Dining rooms that serve as many as thirty to forty residents are just as desirable to consumers as dining rooms that serve as few as sixteen residents. Older adults responded very favorably to cove lighting that provides indirect artificial light, sheer curtains that diffuse natural light, tablecloths and carpeting that minimize reflected glare, and color contrast between tables and floors and tabletops and table settings.*

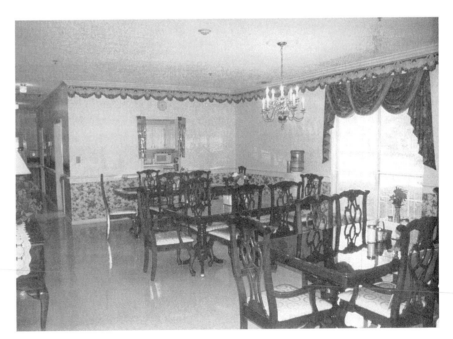

Figure 8.3. *Although traditional tables and chairs are familiar housing cues, the dark wood and the reflected glare from the tabletops drew negative reactions from older adults.*

sumers' perceptions. As a result, separate, well-defined living rooms or living rooms that integrated circulation along the perimeter to facilitate the previewing of a space without interrupting activities within were both acceptable to older adults and family members. In contrast, circulation routes within dining rooms, as in figure 8.4, or adjacent circulation routes that provided views into dining rooms, as in figure 8.5, were less desirable. Both groups of consumers mentioned that they did not want to be viewed by others negotiating hallways and disliked the idea of being on display while eating. Thus, they desired well-defined, separate dining rooms.

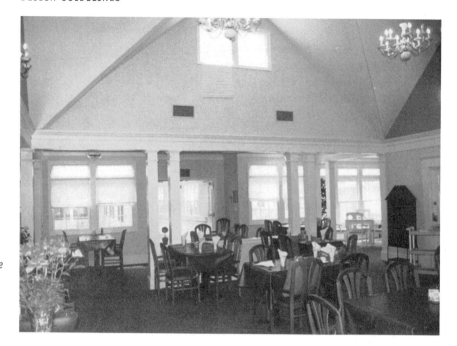

Figure 8.4. *Consumers believed they would be on display while eating if circulation was incorporated in a dining room. Older adults also believe that the chandeliers are positioned too high above the tabletops to be useful; the dark tablecloths, furniture, and carpeting provide little contrast; and the chairs are hard and uncomfortable.*

Caring Cues

Provide Small Table Groupings to Enhance Interaction. Different table shapes and sizes offer various advantages. Square tables, typically for four people, give occupants a more clearly defined territory than do round tables. When square tables are grouped together, they can accommodate a range of people. Round tables are easier to navigate around, since they do not have sharp corners. They typically seat four to ten people. There is a greater possibility for multiple conversations at one table when the group exceeds six people. Oval and rectangular tables provide more tabletop area but space people at greater distances from each other.

Both older adults and family members viewed square and round tables for four people favorably. Smaller table groupings not only enhance human scale but also offer greater opportunities for conversation and facilitate interaction. Tables for six people were viewed less favorably. Long tables or square tables that were grouped together, such as the ones in figure 8.6, drew negative reactions and suggested to the majority of consumers that dining was taking place in a banquet hall or cafeteria.

Avoid Maintenance-free Table Settings. Care can also be exhibited through maintenance. Some assisted living dining rooms included table settings that involved little maintenance. For example, vinyl or plastic tablecloths, glass tabletops over tablecloths, and tables without tablecloths can be easily wiped after meals. Linen tablecloths must be laundered. Plastic cups and glasses, plastic utensils, and paper napkins can be easily thrown away. Silverware and glassware must be cleaned, and linen napkins require laundering. The use of vinyl tablecloths and glass tabletops suggested to family members that older users of the dining room

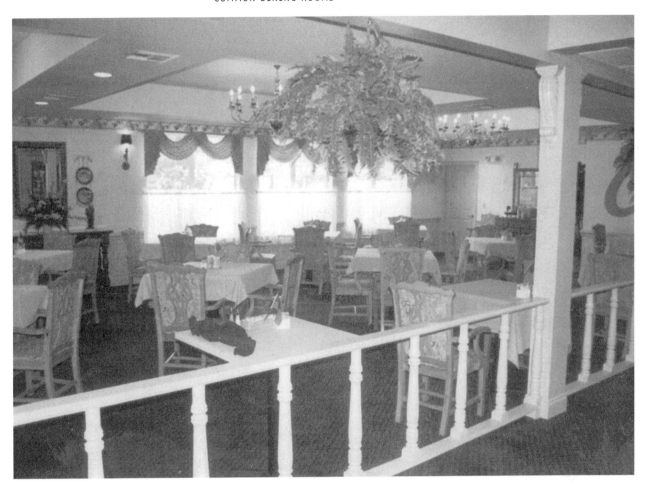

Figure 8.5. *Adjacent circulation routes that provide views into dining rooms are undesirable. Consumers preferred separate dining rooms. Sheer curtains that cover the lower half of windows help to control glare and maintain views at the same time. Consumers responded favorably to real plants, such as the ones in this dining room.*

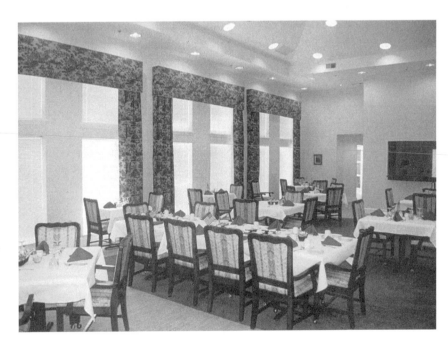

Figure 8.6. *Long tables or square tables grouped together evoke images of cafeterias and banquet halls and suggest that the dining room will be difficult to negotiate and access. Recessed downlighting positioned high above tabletops drew negative reactions from older adults.*

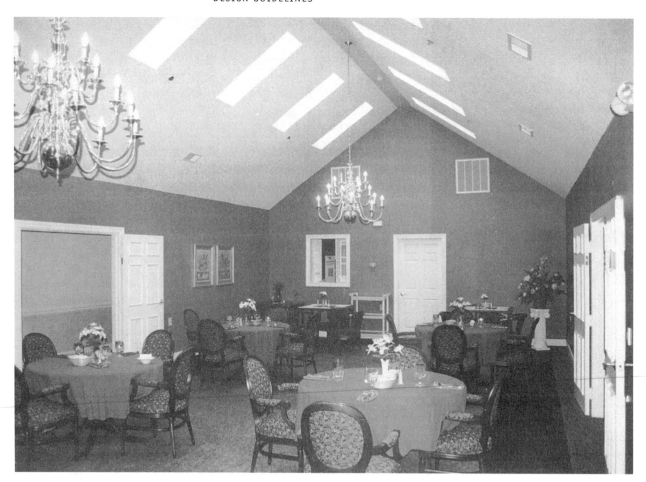

Figure 8.7. *The dining room walls are a medium tone of pink or coral. Although many might find the color garish, older adults favorably rated rooms with bold colors. The skylights near the ceiling ridge provide indirect natural light and help to reduce glare. Although chandeliers provide little usable light, their proximity to the tabletops suggested to older adults that artificial lighting levels would be high in the room. The padded chair backs, seats, and arms were considered very comfortable.*

would be treated like children with messy eating habits. Family members also believed that disposable dinnerware was used for the convenience of staff to save time and costs. Although older adults did not express similar concerns, linen tablecloths and napkins, silverware, and glassware are recommended.

Emphasize Bold Colors. As with interior entries and living rooms, many of the dining rooms that integrated bright, bold colors were considered cheerful, while dark colors were strongly disliked. In particular, older adults were drawn to brightly colored walls that many might find garish. The dining room walls in figure 8.7 are a medium tone of pink or coral. The blue chairs and tables with cloths are easy to identify against the walls. Similarly, the pink upholstered chairs and white tablecloths stand out against the turquoise blue walls in figure 8.8. Because of changes in color perception that accompany old age, bold colors may be needed to stimulate and compensate for sensory losses. Contrasting colors between walls and furniture also improve usability, making it easier for older adults to see the dining room environment. This will be discussed in more detail later in the chapter.

Human Scale

Explore Both Small and Large Spaces. The scale of the dining room in an assisted living building is affected by the ceiling height and the amount of floor area. The amount of floor area needed is usually determined by the number of residents who will be served and the number of seatings offered at each meal. Buildings may include one larger dining room that can accommodate all of the residents in a single seating or one smaller dining room that can accommodate fewer residents in two different seatings. Buildings with two or more smaller dining rooms can serve small groups of residents at the same time. Multiple dining rooms can also minimize distances from resident units when they are placed throughout the building. Research has indicated that decentralized, smaller dining rooms are beneficial in nursing homes with residents with dementia. Schwarz, Chaudhury, Brent, Cooney, Dunne, and Bostick (2001) found that smaller dining rooms for eight to ten residents provide more opportunities for conversations between staff and residents, yield greater staff satisfaction, are less noisy, and result in fewer disruptive behaviors among residents. The amount of floor area is also determined by the arrangement of spaces. The floor area will be greater if the dining room is part of an open plan that includes a kitchen and a family or living room. In dementia care settings, a therapeutic kitchen

Figure 8.8. The pink upholstered chairs and white tablecloths stand out against the turquoise-blue walls. The padded chairs with arm supports are considered comfortable, but the furniture is spaced too closely together, which makes it difficult to negotiate the room.

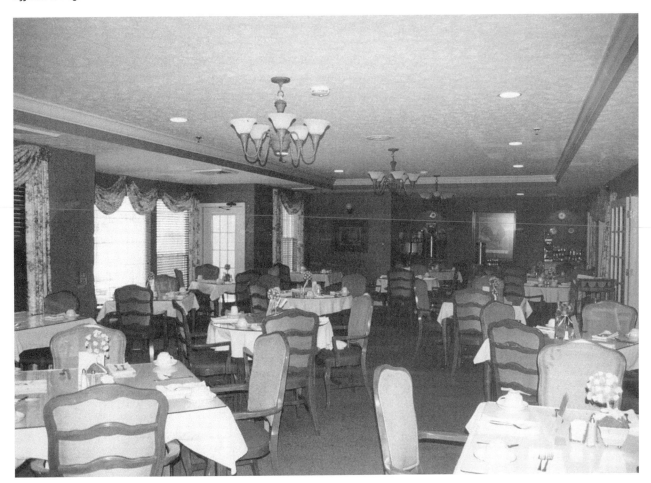

is sometimes part of the dining room and can be used to support activities programming and food service systems (Marsden, Meehan, and Calkins, 2001, 2002).

The assisted living dining rooms included in the research that serves as a basis for this book consisted of both large and small spaces specifically designated for dining. None of the dining rooms included kitchens or family rooms, since such examples were not encountered during the environmental sampling process. An adjacent kitchen was visible from the dining room through a small wall opening in some cases, and some dining rooms were open to circulation routes. Dining rooms with smaller floor areas (serving as few as sixteen residents), as in figure 8.7, and dining rooms with larger floor areas (serving as many as thirty to forty residents), as in figure 8.2, were equally favored by both older adults and family members as long as they provided familiar housing cues and facilitated usability. Larger dining rooms that served greater numbers of people evoked images of restaurants, but consumers felt that this was acceptable for a group living arrangement. Both low and high ceiling heights were also rated favorably by consumers. Even though older adults favored a low ceiling height in interior entries and living rooms, a high ceiling height was desirable in dining rooms if it accommodated clerestory windows or skylights that provided indirect light. Indirect lighting improves usability and will be discussed in more detail in the next section.

Usability

Provide Uniform Lighting. Since older eyes adjust more slowly to changes in brightness, uniform ambient or general lighting of an entire dining room is essential. To achieve uniform lighting, lighting levels must be high to minimize shadows and differences between the lightest and darkest parts of a room. Artificial lighting must also be balanced with daylight for uniform brightness during the day (Brawley, 2001). Research has shown that raising light levels in nursing home dining rooms to reduce uneven lighting levels increases the independence and caloric intake of residents with dementia (Brush, 2001; Koss and Gilmore, 1998).

Indirect lighting systems are effective for uniform lighting. With indirect lighting, the majority of light is directed toward the ceiling and upper walls and reflected downward. The lighter the color of the ceiling and upper walls, the more light is reflected and diffused into the space below. Cove lighting is an indirect artificial lighting system in which the light source is shielded by a ledge or recess and distributed over the ceiling. Some pendant fixtures also conceal the light source and direct light up to the ceiling. Wall sconces provide indirect electric lighting by reflecting light onto the walls and the ceiling. They are usually a secondary ambient light source, since they do not generate enough light on their own to illuminate an entire space. When ceilings are higher than eight feet, clerestory windows, high on the wall, and skylights can provide indirect natural light during the day. The exclusive use of indirect lighting can be very flat, and task and accent lighting are sometimes added to a room for interest. Supplemental lighting, however, should not be dramatically brighter than the surrounding area. Noell-Waggoner (2002) noted that the Illuminating Engineering Society of North America (IESNA) recommends a ratio that does not exceed 3 to 1.

Although more difficult to achieve, uniform lighting is also possible in the dining room with direct lighting systems. Direct lighting consists of light that is directed downward. The ceiling is illuminated by light reflected from the floor and furnishings. Recessed lighting, surface-mounted ceiling fixtures, and some pendant fixtures provide direct lighting. Several issues must be taken into account if a direct lighting system is used. First, the ceiling may appear dark if insufficient light is reflected from the floor and furnishings. Second, the spacing of fixtures is usually determined by the ceiling height and the width of the light beam. Many fixtures, evenly spaced throughout the room, are usually necessary for uniform lighting. In a larger space, this can result in row after row of pendants or a ceiling filled with holes to accommodate recessed cans. Third, downlights often provide overlapping beams of light that create hot spots or bright patches in rooms with low ceilings. Downlights are more effective in spaces with high ceilings because hot spots are not as apparent and lighting appears more uniform. A greater distance between the fixture and the table below, however, decreases the overall light level.

Uniform lighting in assisted living dining rooms is very important to older adults. Older persons responded positively to cove lighting, as shown in the dining room in figure 8.2, which provides indirect artificial lighting. They also strongly favored skylights, as shown in figure 8.7, and clerestory windows, as shown in figure 8.9, for indirect natural light. In addition, evenly spaced fixtures that provided uniform direct lighting were well received. For example, older persons reacted positively to the surface-mounted fixtures in the dining room in figure 8.10, even though the fixtures were unfamiliar housing cues and many fixtures lined the ceiling. Although the need for uniform lighting was not salient in family members' perceptions, it is imperative to investigate indirect and direct lighting systems that provide uniform lighting to meet the needs of older adults. In addition, it is important to investigate both artificial and natural lighting systems to accommodate dining at different times of the day.

Reduce Glare. Because of aging-related changes in the eye, older adults are more sensitive to glare. Unshielded light bulbs or sunlight streaming through a window provides direct glare when it is in a person's immediate field of vision. A high contrast between daylight and dim artificial lighting in an interior space also contributes to direct glare. High contrast occurs when windows on a single side of a room create a bright area. Objects in front of the window are then seen as dark silhouettes. A bright window that contrasts against a darker wall or a skylight against a darker vaulted ceiling will also be seen as bright spots that

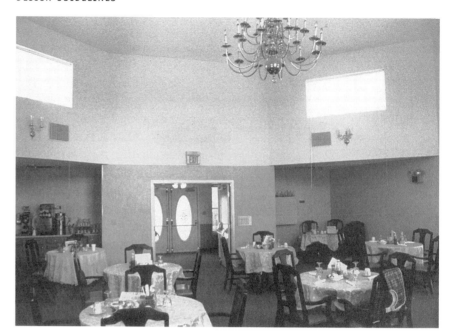

Figure 8.9. *Clerestory windows, as in this dining room, provide indirect natural light and help to reduce glare. Clerestory windows on two sides help to balance light throughout the room.*

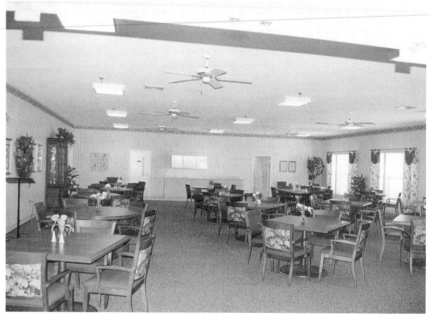

Figure 8.10. *Older persons reacted positively to the uniform lighting provided by the evenly spaced downlighting in this dining room, even though the fixtures are unfamiliar housing cues. Older persons also believed that the light levels are high because of the short distance between the fixtures and the tabletops. Tables that are spaced far apart facilitate accessibility and private conversations during mealtime. In addition, real plants throughout the room and flower arrangements in the center of tables are connections to nature.*

cause direct glare. Reflected glare results when intense light bounces off of a light-colored or shiny, smooth surface into the eye.

Direct glare can be controlled with clerestory windows and skylights. Older adults commented that such openings would not blind them and would make it easier to navigate the dining room and see the food on their tables. High windows and skylights increase light levels and reduce glare at the same time by balancing natural and artificial light. Several strategies can be used with clerestory windows and skylights to create an even brighter space with less glare. First, light can be brought through clerestory windows on two different sides of the din-

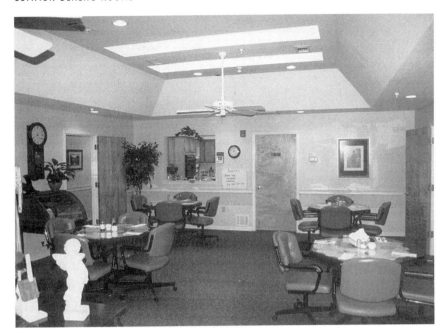

Figure 8.11. *The splayed ceiling trays help to reflect light entering through the skylights. The proximity of the skylights to the edges of the room also helps to illuminate the walls.*

ing room, as in figure 8.9, to balance light throughout the room. Second, skylights near the ridge of a ceiling, as in figure 8.7, allow light entering from one side of a white, vaulted ceiling to flow down the opposite side. Splayed ceiling trays, as in figure 8.11, help to reflect light entering through skylights. Since the skylights are close to the edge of the dining room, the light also illuminates the walls. The soffit that encircles the room helps to prevent the ceiling from being too high for human scale. The size and positioning of all openings should be considered in relation to the orientation of the sun.

The elimination of direct glare was so important to older adults that they rated dining rooms with clerestory windows or skylights favorably even when the rooms did not include windows at eye level with views to the outdoors. Window views are important features of naturalness in interior entries and living rooms. Windows at eye level were more desirable to older adults when they included sheer curtains that diffuse light, as shown in figure 8.2, or shades that filter light. Sheer curtains that cover the lower half of windows, as depicted in figure 8.5, or shades that can be activated from the top down or bottom up can control glare and maintain views at the same time.

The elimination of reflected glare was important to older adults, too. Carpeting and matte table finishes, as shown in the dining room in figure 8.12, were favorable features. Tablecloths, a familiar housing cue and a sign of care, also helped to reduce reflected glare. In contrast, resilient flooring, such as sheet vinyl and vinyl composition tile sealed with polish, hardwood floors with a polyurethane finish, and Pergo laminated flooring with a reflective coating provided undesirable shiny surfaces. Tables with polished or glass tops were also undesirable (see figs. 8.3 and 8.13). Family members were less concerned with glare and its affect on the ability of consumers to function in dining rooms. In

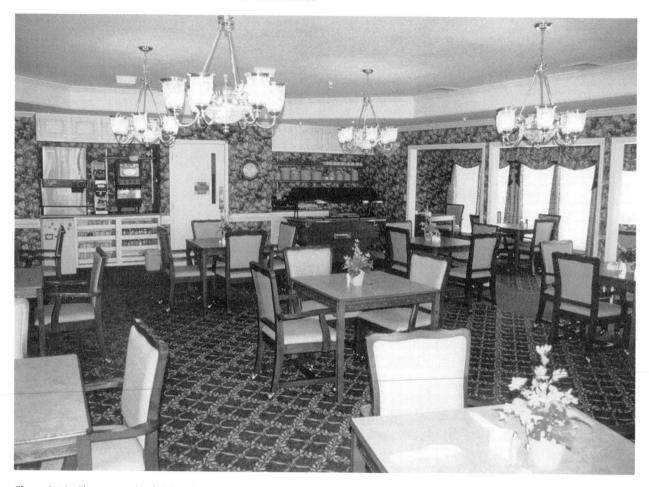

Figure 8.12. *The matte table finish and carpeting help to reduce reflected glare in this dining room. The pendants are close to the tabletops, which suggested to older adults that lighting levels would be high. Older adults also considered padded chair seats and backs comfortable and responded favorably to the flower arrangements on the tables.*

fact, they favored hardwood floors as features of naturalness. To meet the vision needs of older adults, avoid shiny surfaces and use matte finishes.

Provide Lighting Fixtures Close to Tables. As stated previously, the distance between light fixtures and tabletops can affect the level and uniformity of lighting. Older adults favorably rated dining rooms with light fixtures positioned close to tabletops. It seems that they believed that small distances would result in higher lighting levels and facilitate eating. For example, fixtures mounted on a low ceiling (fig. 8.10), pendants suspended a short distance from a low ceiling (fig. 8.12), and chandeliers suspended a great distance from a high ceiling (fig. 8.7) drew positive reactions. Even though chandeliers provide little usable light, older adults still responded favorably to them when they were positioned close to tabletops. In contrast, the chandeliers in the vaulted dining room in figure 8.4 and the recessed downlighting in figure 8.6 are positioned high above the tables and were considered less useful. Family members placed greater emphasis on fixtures as decorative elements and were less concerned with the distance between fixtures and tables. To meet the needs of older adults, place fixtures with shielded light sources close to tabletops to facilitate eating. They should also be sup-

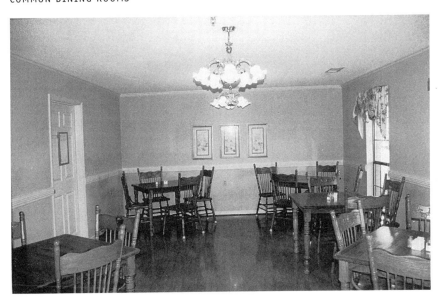

Figure 8.13. *Hardwood floors with a polyurethane finish create undesirable shiny surfaces. Chairs without padded seats and backs are considered uncomfortable.*

plemented with indirect lighting systems, as previously discussed. In addition, fixtures should include familiar cues to satisfy family members' concerns.

Use Color Contrast on Tabletops and Chair Upholstery. Low vision makes it difficult for older adults to locate tables and chairs in a dining room, to identify the edges of dishes and utensils, and to find food on their plates. Research has shown that contrast between the plate and the table or place setting increases caloric intake (Brush, 2001). Color contrast between tables and floors, tables and chairs, and tables and table settings is recommended. In particular, older adults responded favorably to dining rooms with light-colored tablecloths that stood out against darker chairs and floors. For example, the dining room in figure 8.2 includes a white tablecloth, peach-colored napkins, dark carpeting, and upholstered chairs with a medium tone of color and dark wood edges. Dark wood tables without tablecloths and dark wood chairs with dark upholstery, as in figure 8.1, drew negative reactions. Similarly, dark blue tablecloths and dark wood chairs against dark flooring provided little contrast in the dining room in figure 8.4.

Provide Comfortable Dining Room Chairs. Both older adults and family members responded favorably to chairs with padding, upholstery, and arm supports. Consumers believed that padded seats and backs with upholstery would be comfortable and soft on the skin (see figs. 8.8 and 8.12). They also believed that chair arms could be used as a resting place for people's arms and as support when rising from a seated position. The chairs in the dining room in figure 8.7 were considered particularly comfortable. The chair seat, back, and arms are all padded. In contrast, the chairs in figures 8.4 and 8.13 were considered hard and uncomfortable.

Consumers expressed both positive and negative reactions to chairs with casters or wheels. Sometimes the front legs of chairs include cast-

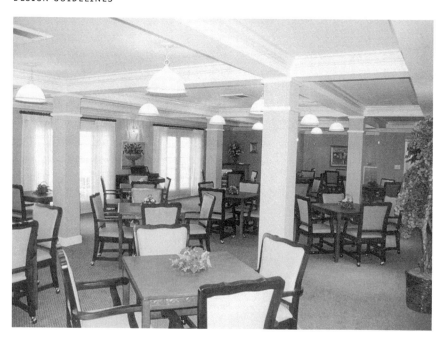

Figure 8.14. *Architectural features, such as columns, used to divide a larger dining room can be intrusive and negatively affect the ability of older adults to navigate the space.*

ers, as in figure 8.6. In other instances, casters are added to the back legs of chairs (see fig. 8.12). It has been assumed that casters make it easier for residents to pull up to and push away from a table on their own. When unsteady residents rise from a chair, however, casters may make the chair unstable. Thus, casters may be appropriate only for higher-functioning residents (Briller, Proffitt, Perez, Calkins, and Marsden, 2001). Additional research is needed in this area to determine whether casters are appropriate for certain segments of the older population.

Provide Room to Navigate around Furniture. Older adults favored dining rooms with table groupings spaced far apart (see figs. 8.10 and 8.12) and disliked those with furniture grouped too closely together (see fig. 8.8). The ability to navigate around furniture is an important concern for older adults, especially if they must use wheelchairs, walkers, or canes. In addition, tables that are spaced farther apart assured older adults that they could carry on mealtime conversations privately and would not have to fear eavesdropping. Older adults also found architectural features, such as columns, used to break up larger dining rooms into smaller areas intrusive. They believed the columns in the dining room in figure 8.14 would interfere with their attempts to ambulate around furniture. Family members, however, were less concerned with space around furniture for easy movement or private conversations and even expressed a preference for tables spaced closer together. To meet the needs of older adults, space furniture farther apart.

Naturalness

Utilize Windows and Skylights for Natural Light and Views. Consumers favored window views to the outdoors because they provide connections to nature, the time of day, the season of the year, and changes in weather. Windows can, however, also be sources of glare. As discussed

98

previously, the provision of windows at eye level in dining rooms is not as important to older adults when clerestory windows or skylights are present. Windows at eye level are more acceptable if light is diffused with sheer curtains or shades. Whether windows are at eye level to offer views or are located high on walls to reduce glare, natural light in the dining room is recommended. Sunlight is a connection to nature. Artificial light can never simulate the intensity, color, and warmth of natural light.

Provide Real Indoor Plants and Flowers. Real plants and flowers are strong connections to nature and provide opportunities for older adults to care for something that is alive. Both older adults and family members were attracted to flower arrangements centered on dining room tables, as in figures 8.10 and 8.12, and plants located throughout the space, as shown in figures 8.5 and 8.10.

Conclusion

The studies that serve as a foundation for this book indicate that consumers do not always perceive assisted living buildings as supportive and friendly. As discussed in chapter 3, the literature and popular press are filled with numerous examples of critically acclaimed buildings that are designed in ways that do not support people's well-being. This has largely been attributed to the efforts of well-meaning designers who are apparently unaware of user needs. In assisted living, there has been a movement toward the delivery of services based on the needs and wishes articulated by residents, but there has been little attempt to do the same with the design of the physical environment.

This book is about the humanistic design of assisted living for consumers. Humanistic design entails consumer input. Older people who occupy assisted living buildings and family members who periodically visit should have a say about the environment. This is possible when consumers are asked about their needs and their perceptions of environments in the context of scientific research. Research-based information, translated into design guidelines that are easily applied by those without a research background, can be used to supplement intuitions and help architects and designers make more informed design decisions. Architects and designers are then more likely to create humane buildings that cultivate well-being and support consumers' abilities to function effectively.

Drawing from the research that serves as a basis for this book, the final chapter summarizes the design needs of older residents of assisted living and of family members, taking into account their similarities and differences. These consumer needs are discussed in relation to the conceptual framework for humanistic design that has been used throughout the chapters on design guidelines. The final chapter also summarizes in tables the specific design recommendations for building exteriors, interior entries, common living rooms, and common dining rooms and reconciles differences between the consumer groups. The tables are intended to provide a quick checklist for those involved in developing assisted living buildings.

A Summary of Consumer Needs

Based on in-depth interviews with residents of assisted living, Frank (1999, 2002) concluded that assisted living can never be "home" for older people because of the complexity of the phenomenon of home. Assisted living buildings can be designed, however, in ways that are more humane and that provide opportunities for consumers to derive enjoyment from architecture and to function effectively. Throughout

101

this book, several constructs that are central to the humanistic design of assisted living have been stressed: familiar housing cues, protective enclosure, caring cues, human scale, usability, and naturalness. These constructs may not guarantee humane design, but architects and designers are more likely to create humane assisted living buildings for older adults and family members if they use them. Similarly, architects and designers may be able to apply the design guidelines to other housing options for older adults, such as buildings for independent living and nursing homes.

Familiar Housing Cues

Both older adults and family members reacted favorably to cues that reference the single-family house. Porches, porticos, sloped roofs, gables, window shutters, diverse window shapes and sizes, fireplaces, a formal residential décor in the dining room, and an informal décor in the living room are examples. Unfamiliar housing cues such as the porte-cochere, flat roofs, metal front doors, freestanding flagpoles, uniform window sizes, an information desk with a large built-in counter or workstation, certain holiday decorations, lack of detail, and bare interior walls drew negative reactions from both groups of consumers.

Despite the similarities, family members placed greater emphasis on familiar housing cues while older adults viewed building exteriors and interior spaces more in terms of usability. For example, family members viewed pedestrian covered walkways such as canopies unfavorably because they included an unfamiliar housing cue. In contrast, older adults were willing to overlook the unfamiliar housing cue because it provided shelter and would make it easier for them to walk from the car to the front door if it was raining. When a cue became too unfamiliar or over-sized, however, as with a porte-cochere, the need for familiar housing cues became more important to older adults than usability. Similarly, family members placed a great emphasis on traditional dining room furniture with dark wood, while older adults felt that dark wood was difficult to see and contributed to a dark space. Family members were also drawn to dining room chandeliers as a familiar cue even when they were positioned high above tables and provided little usable light for older adults while eating.

Protective Enclosure

Layers of enclosure from the site edge to the building interior and transitional areas between public and private were important to both older adults and family members. In addition, both groups considered balconies that are partially enclosed or inset into the building safer than ones that project beyond the building. Visible rooflines suggested protective enclosure, but older adults did not like the idea of living within the volume of a roof. Dormers implied uncomfortable and unusable attic space to older adults but were familiar housing cues to family members.

In general, older adults stressed the need for protective enclosure with sheltered exterior entries and interior spaces more than did family members. Specifically, older adults desired some shelter along a walkway to the building entrance. They also favored interior entries that were well defined as separate rooms with little visual access to other spaces. Family members did not mind open interior entries that were visually and spatially connected to adjacent rooms or spaces on upper floors. In addition, older adults desired well-defined dining rooms that did not include circulation routes through the space or adjacent hallways with views into the space. Older adults did not want to feel as if they were on display while eating.

Caring Cues

Attention to details such as quoins, lintels, and other ornamentation on the outside and inside of the building suggests that care is evident. Both groups of consumers were attracted to signs of human occupancy such as open windows and window treatments and outdoor seating. A small desk with a friendly greeter in the interior entry and entrance doors with glazing are also welcoming features. The need for physical attributes that communicate care was particularly evident in living rooms. Small seating arrangements that encourage social exchange; televisions, radios, pianos, bookshelves, and game tables that support activity choices; separate activity areas that permit occupants to pursue activities simultaneously; and bright, cheerful colors that animate the environment were desirable to older adults and family members.

Care can be also exhibited through maintenance. Both groups felt that linen tablecloths and napkins, silverware, and glassware on dining room tables suggested care. Vinyl tablecloths, plastic utensils and glasses, and paper napkins suggested that staff convenience was more important. Both groups felt that buildings and the surrounding landscape should be fresh and maintained reasonably well. Perfectly manicured landscapes and sterile rooms were less desirable. Family members favored older buildings as familiar living arrangements for older adults. Older adults, however, felt that older buildings implied maintenance and accessibility problems.

Human Scale

Both older adults and family members were drawn to decorative features and smaller parts of the building that help to minimize the scale of the building façade and interior spaces. Other features such as gables, a variety of rooflines, changes in materials, setbacks, and different window and balcony shapes help to reduce the perceived massiveness of the façade. Small bookcases, small table groupings for four, and somewhat close spacing between furniture help to reduce the scale of interior spaces. In addition, older adults stressed the need for a one-story building height, one-story exterior entries, and lower ceilings in interior entries and living rooms. Higher ceilings were acceptable in dining rooms if they accommodated clerestory windows or skylights that provided indirect natural light. Larger dining rooms that accommodate as many as thirty to forty people and resemble restaurants were also acceptable for a group living arrangement. In contrast, building and ceiling height as well as spatial volume were less important to family members.

Usability

Older adults viewed exterior entries and interior spaces in terms of how well they might be able to use and access the rooms based on their age-related impairments. In particular, they favored exterior entries on grade and windows that permitted seated people to view the outside. Within interior entries, they desired a clear path from the front door and enough room to navigate around central focal points, level changes of floor material, and carpeting or flooring with matte finishes to reduce glare. Adequate spacing between couches and chairs and furniture with padded but firm seating in living rooms was important. Overstuffed furniture or furniture with loose pillows for back support was less desirable. The usability of a space was particularly important in dining rooms where older adults spend a great deal of time. Clerestory windows and skylights help to provide uniform natural light and reduce glare, sheer curtains and shades diffuse natural light from windows at eye level, and cove lighting provides indirect artificial lighting. Adequate spacing between table groupings facilitates accessibility and private conversations. In contrast, usability was much less salient in family members' perceptions.

Naturalness

Both older adults and family members were drawn to buildings that reference nature. Direct connections to lush landscaping, interior plants and flowers, and natural light as well as indirect connections provided by window views and building materials such as wood and brick are desirable. When nature is used in an artificial way in interior spaces with fake plants or materials such as green carpeting and wallpaper that simulates brick, perceptions were inconsistent with expectations for how a space should appear and function.

Summary of Design Guidelines

Guidelines that consider similarities in perception between older adults and family members and reconcile differences between the consumer groups were developed in relation to the conceptual framework. These are discussed in detail in chapters 5, 6, 7, and 8 and are summarized in the tables in this chapter. Table 1 presents summary guidelines for building façades and exterior entries. The guidelines for interior entries are summarized in table 2, while tables 3 and 4 address living rooms and dining rooms, respectively. As noted in the introduction, the design guidelines do not cover individual resident units, hallways, outdoor areas, or back-of-house spaces. Empirical research that focuses on these spaces is needed in the future.

Table 1 Design Guidelines: Building Exteriors

Familiar Housing Cues
- View the porte-cochere as an extension of the front façade rather than as an imposing front addition.
- Consider separate vehicular and pedestrian entries.
- Explore variations of the portico and the porch.
- Reference gables, sloped roofs, window shutters, front lawns, gutters, downspouts, cresting, and finials.
- Consider windows and balconies that vary in size and shape.
- Place common areas toward the front of the building if diverse window shapes and sizes for individual units present marketing challenges.

Protective Enclosure
- Porticos and porches that project beyond the building edge can provide shelter from the car to the entry and sheltered seating at the entry.
- Provide some enclosure with railings or half-walls at the porch edge.
- Provide layers of enclosure and transition with fences, front lawns, porches, balconies, foundation shrubs, vegetation on walls, and visible rooflines.
- Partially enclose balconies by insetting them into the building or projecting walls beyond the façade.
- Consider bow and bay windows.
- Use dormers that include air vents rather than windows that imply unusable attic space.

Caring Cues
- Make sure shrubs are well tended and do not block window views.
- Provide seating, arranged in small groupings, at the entry.
- Include glazed entry doors, fanlights, sidelights, and transom windows to provide glimpses of the interior.
- Emphasize signs of human occupancy with walkable sidewalks, open and drawn window treatments, and seating.
- Consider details such as window muntins, quoins, and lintels to suggest careful attention to the act of building.
- Maintain the landscaping and building exterior reasonably well.
- Consider the adaptive reuse of older buildings on a case-by-case basis.
- Consider light colors for façades and contrasting colors for front doors, shutters, and details.

Human Scale
- Position the front door close to the driveway.
- Pay attention to details such as window muntins, quoins, and lintels.
- When economies of scale permit, limit buildings to one story for scale and accessibility.
- Consider one-story entries.
- Reduce the perceived massing of façades with cross gables, a variety of roof lines, changes in materials, setbacks, and different window and balcony shapes.
- Pay attention to smaller parts of the building, including foundation shrubs, potted plants, low fencing, building materials (thin wood siding, brick, roof tile), entry columns and pilasters, fanlights, sidelights, and detailing (porch and balcony railings, window trim, lintels or arches, shutters, string courses, quoins, bargeboard, cornices).
- Consider tall, vertical windows with muntins that divide the glass into panes.

Usability
- Consider porches that are level with the ground.
- When porches are above grade, integrate ramps and railings into the porch design.
- Make sure unit balconies are deep enough to accommodate outdoor furniture and activities.
- Provide outdoor chairs with arm rests.
- Make sure windows permit views to the outdoors for people seated inside.

Naturalness
- Consider small front lawns.
- Use wood and brick building materials where contextually appropriate.
- Preserve mature trees by locating and configuring the building around existing trees.
- Add well-tended, lush landscaping including foundation shrubs, potted plants, and flowers.

Table 2 Design Guidelines: Interior Entries

Familiar Housing Cues
- An information desk should be a movable piece of furniture such as a writing table, secretary, console, or bureau rather than a built-in counter or large executive desk that resembles a workstation.
- Reference the fireplace and residential décor including artwork, window treatments, table lamps, and chandeliers.
- Use holiday decorations cautiously, making sure that they are not childlike.
- Make sure interior entry spaces are consistent with how the foyer of a single-family house would look and function.

Protective Enclosure
- Create a well-defined space that is a separate room with a lower ceiling and some visual access to other spaces through wall openings.

Caring Cues
- Provide a friendly information desk so that a staff member can greet people and offer assistance.
- Provide a small seating area consisting of two or three armchairs or upholstered chairs rather than large couches.
- Use bright, cheerful colors, as opposed to dark colors, for window treatments and floor coverings.

Human Scale
- Lower ceilings and explore ceiling variations (tray, vault, cathedral, dome, dropped) to add spatial diversity.
- Accentuate decorative moldings on ceilings and walls, where surfaces meet, and around openings and fireplaces.

Usability
- Integrate cove lighting into the ceiling architecture.
- Keep the path from the front door clear and provide enough room to navigate around central focal points.
- To reduce glare from windows and door glazing, use carpeting and flooring with matte finishes and investigate sun-control devices that are familiar housing cues.
- Make sure all transitions between different floor materials are level.

Naturalness
- Consider doors with glazing, fanlights, sidelights, and transom windows that provide views to landscaping, wildlife, the sky, and outdoor activities.
- Create a colorful focal point with live flower arrangements on center tables, fireplace mantels, and information desks.

Table 3   Design Guidelines: Living Rooms

Familiar Housing Cues
- Provide a less formal décor based on the furniture style and arrangement, upholstery color and pattern, window treatments, lighting fixtures, and finishes.
- Reference the fireplace, shelves for books or ornaments, and residential décor including artwork, window treatments, and table lamps.

Protective Enclosure
- Consider living rooms that are separate rooms, or integrate circulation to allow consumers to preview the space.

Caring Cues
- Arrange furniture around a focal point that is a familiar housing cue, such as a fireplace, window, piece of furniture, artwork, decorative rug, or flower arrangement.
- If there is more than one focal point, make sure they work together or divide the room into two or more areas to minimize competition between foci.
- Incorporate features such as televisions, radios, pianos, bookshelves, game tables, and seating that support activity choices.
- Consider separate activity areas so that activities can be pursued simultaneously.
- Use bright, cheerful colors, as opposed to dark colors, for upholstery and floor coverings.

Human Scale
- Consider smaller floor areas, lower ceiling heights, and somewhat close spacing between furniture.
- Focus on small-scale elements such as decorative moldings, divided lights in windows, and ornaments on tables, shelves, and fireplace mantels.
- Consider multiple, smaller bookcases or shelves rather than one large wall unit.

Usability
- Make sure furniture is spaced close enough to facilitate conversation but distant enough to allow older adults to navigate the space.
- Provide couches and chairs with padded but firm seating and backs as well as arm supports, and avoid overstuffed furniture with loose pillows.

Naturalness
- Consider wood for bookcases or shelves.
- Make sure living rooms include windows for natural light and outdoor views.
- Provide real plants and flowers that are within easy reach and can be cared for by consumers.

Table 4   Design Guidelines: Dining Rooms

Familiar Housing Cues
- Provide a formal décor based on the furniture style, lighting fixtures, window treatments, table settings, and finishes.
- Reference hutches, cabinets, or breakfronts for displaying china and glassware, sideboards, buffets, servers, chandeliers, window treatments, and artwork.

Protective Enclosure
- Consider well-defined, separate dining rooms so that older adults do not feel like they are being watched by others negotiating circulation routes.

Caring Cues
- Provide small tables for four to facilitate interaction, and avoid grouping several tables together.
- Consider linen tablecloths and napkins, silverware, and glassware, and avoid vinyl or plastic tablecloths, plastic cups and glasses, plastic utensils, and paper napkins.
- Emphasize bold and cheerful wall colors.

Human Scale
- Explore spaces that include both smaller floor areas (serving as few as 16 residents) and larger floor areas (serving as many as 30–40 residents).
- Consider low ceiling heights.
- Consider higher ceiling heights if they accommodate clerestory windows or skylights that provide indirect light.
- Use ceiling soffits around the perimeter of the room to lower high ceilings.

Usability
- Provide uniform artificial lighting with indirect systems such as cove lighting or direct systems such as evenly spaced pendants or surface-mounted fixtures.
- Provide uniform natural lighting with clerestory windows and skylights that provide indirect light.
- Use clerestory windows and skylights to increase light levels, balance natural and artificial light, and reduce glare.
- Consider clerestory windows on two different sides of the dining room, skylights near the ceiling ridge and the walls, and splayed ceiling trays to create brighter spaces with reduced glare.
- Use sheer curtains or shades that can be activated from the top down or bottom up for windows at eye level to control glare and maintain views.
- Use tablecloths and matte table finishes rather than polished tabletops to minimize reflected glare.
- Consider carpeting rather than shiny hardwood floors, laminated flooring, or sheet vinyl to reduce reflected glare.
- Position light fixtures close to tabletops to enhance perceptions of increased lighting.
- Use color contrast between tables and floors, tables and chairs, and tables and table settings.
- Consider chairs with padded seats and backs, upholstery, and arm supports.
- Use casters cautiously on chairs for higher-functioning residents.
- Provide sufficient spacing between table groupings to facilitate accessibility and private table conversations.
- Avoid architectural features such as columns that divide the space and affect accessibility.

Naturalness
- Utilize windows and skylights for natural light and views, but make sure glare is controlled.
- Provide real indoor plants and flower arrangements on tabletops.

REFERENCES

Alexander, C., Ishikawa, S., Silverstein, M., Jacobson, M., Fiksdahl-King, I., and Angel, S. (1977). *A pattern language.* New York: Oxford University Press.

American Association of Retired Persons (AARP). (1996). *Understanding senior housing in the next century: Survey of consumer preferences, concerns and needs.* Washington, DC: AARP.

American Association of Retired Persons (AARP). (2000). *Fixing to stay: A national survey on housing and home modifications.* Washington, DC: AARP.

American Institute of Architecture Students (AIAS). (2002). *The redesign of studio culture: A report of the AIAS Studio Culture Task Force.* Washington, DC: AIAS.

Anthony, K. (1991). *Design juries on trial: The renaissance of the design studio.* New York: Van Nostrand Reinhold.

Arenson, M. C. (1998, June). Not in our backyard. *Nursing Homes Long Term Care Management,* 47(6), 24–30.

Assisted Living Federation of America (ALFA). (1998). *The assisted living industry: An overview—1998.* Fairfax, VA: PriceWaterhouseCoopers.

Assisted Living Federation of America (ALFA). (2000). *ALFA's overview of the industry.* Fairfax, VA: PriceWaterhouseCoopers and National Investment Center.

Assisted Living Federation of America (ALFA). (2001). *ALFA's 2001 overview of the industry: A supplement report.* Fairfax, VA: PriceWaterhouseCoopers and National Investment Center.

Assisted Living Workgroup. (2003). *Assuring quality in assisted living: Guidelines for federal and state policy, state regulation, and operations.* Washington, DC: National Center for Assisted Living and American Association of Homes & Services for the Aging.

Association of Collegiate Schools of Architecture (ACSA). (2004). *Architectural education.* www.acsa-arch.org/architecturalEd.html; accessed August 22, 2004.

Barry, C. D. (1999). *The experience of moving into an assisted living facility: A Heideggerian hermeneutical phenomenological inquiry.* Unpublished doctoral dissertation, University of Miami.

Becker, F. (1977). *Housing messages.* Stroudsburg, PA: Dowden Hutchinson & Ross.

Bentley, L., Sabo, S., and Waye, A. E. (2003). *Assisted living state regulatory review 2003.* Washington, DC: National Center for Assisted Living.

Berlowitz, D. R., Du, W., Kazis, L., and Lewis, S. (1995). Health-related quality of life of nursing home residents: Difference in patient and provider perceptions. *Journal of the American Geriatrics Society,* 43, 799–802.

Bonvissuto, K. (2003, May 5). Rethinking the retirement community. *Crain's Cleveland Business,* 24(18), 15.

Boyer, E., and Mitgang, L. (1996). *Building community: A new future for architectural education and practice.* Princeton, NJ: Carnegie Foundation for the Advancement of Teaching.

Brawley, E. C. (1997). *Designing for Alzheimer's disease: Strategies for creating better care environments.* New York: John Wiley & Sons.

Brawley, E. C. (2001). Environmental design for Alzheimer's disease: A quality of life issue. *Aging and Mental Health,* 5(Suppl. 1), S79–S83.

Briller, S. H., Proffitt, M. A., Perez, K. R., and Calkins, M. P. (2001). *Understanding the environment through the aging senses,* Vol. 1 in M. P. Calkins, *Creating successful dementia care settings* (series). Baltimore: Health Professions Press.

Briller, S. H., Proffitt, M. A., Perez, K. R., Calkins, M. P., and Marsden, J. P. (2001). *Maximizing cognitive and functional abilities,* Vol. 2 in M. P. Calkins, *Creating successful dementia care settings* (series). Baltimore: Health Professions Press.

Brown, G., and Gifford, R. (2001). Architects predict lay evaluations of large contemporary buildings: Whose conceptual properties? *Journal of Environmental Psychology,* 21, 93–99.

Brummett, W. (1997). *The essence of home: Design solutions for assisted living housing.* New York: Van Nostrand Reinhold.

Brush, J. (2001). *Improving dining for people with dementia.* Milwaukee: Center for Architecture & Planning Research, University of Wisconsin–Milwaukee.

Calkins, M. P. (1988). *Design for dementia: Planning environments for the elderly and the confused.* Owings Mills, MD: National Health Publishing.

Calkins, M. P. (2001a). Special care units and the environment: Advances of the past decade. *Alzheimer's Care Quarterly,* 2(3), 41–48.

Calkins, M. P. (2001b). The physical and social environment of the person with Alzheimer's disease. *Aging and Mental Health,* 5(Suppl. 1), S74–S78.

Camp, C. J., West, R. L., and Poon, L. W. (1989). Recruitment practices for psychological research in gerontology. In M. P. Lawton and A. R. Herzog (Eds.), *Special research methods in gerontology.* Amityville, NY: Baywood Publishing.

Carpman, J. R., and Grant, M. A. (1993). *Design that cares: Planning health facilities for patients and visitors.* Chicago: American Hospital Publishing.

Cinelli, D. J. (1999). Place makes a difference: A case study in assisted living. In B. Schwarz and R. Brent (Eds.), *Aging, autonomy and architecture: Advances in assisted living* (pp. 262–277). Baltimore: Johns Hopkins University Press.

Cohen, U., and Day, K. (1993). *Contemporary environments for people with dementia.* Baltimore: Johns Hopkins University Press.

Cohen, U., and Weisman, G. D. (1991). *Holding on to home: Designing environments for people with dementia.* Baltimore: Johns Hopkins University Press.

Cooper Marcus, C. (1995). *House as a mirror of self: Exploring the deeper meanings of home.* Berkeley, CA: Conari Press.

Corcoran, M., and Gitlin, L. N. (1991). Environmental influences on behavior of the elderly with dementia: Principles for intervention in the home. *Physical and Occupational Therapy in Geriatrics,* 9(3/4), 5–22.

Cuff, D. (1991). *Architecture: The story of practice.* Cambridge: MIT Press.

Day, C. (1990). *Places of the soul: Architecture and environmental design as healing art.* London: Thorsons.

Day, K., and Calkins, M. P. (2002). Design and dementia. In R. B. Bechtel and A. Churchman (Eds.), *Handbook of environmental psychology* (pp. 374–393). New York: John Wiley & Sons.

Day, K., Carreon, D., and Stump, C. (2000). The therapeutic design of environments for people with dementia: A review of the empirical research. *The Gerontologist,* 40(4), 397–416.

Devlin, K. (1990). An examination of architectural interpretation: Architects versus non-architects. *Journal of Architectural and Planning Research,* 7, 235–244.

Devlin, K., and Nasar, J. L. (1989). The beauty and the beast: Some preliminary comparisons of "high" versus "popular" residential architecture and public versus architect judgments of same. *Journal of Environmental Psychology,* 9, 334–344.

Dixon, G., Parshall, P., Pratt, D., Solinger, J., and Young, D. (2001). The foundations of marketing: Referral development and successful strategies. In K. H. Namazi and P. K. Chafetz (Eds.), *Assisted living: Current issues in facility management and resident care* (pp. 65–76). Westport, CT: Auburn House.

Durand, K. T. (2001). An owner's/operator's view of assisted living facilities' development and progress. In K. H. Namazi and P. K. Chafetz (Eds.), *Assisted living: Current issues in facility management and resident care* (pp. 183–191). Westport, CT: Auburn House.

ElderWeb (2004). *LTC backwards and forwards.* www.elderweb.com/default.php?PageID=2806; accessed August 22, 2004.

Elrod, C. L. (2002). *A qualitative analysis of the presence of sense of community, perceived social support, and social participation behaviors in small, rural assisted living facilities.* Unpublished doctoral dissertation, Georgia State University.

Federal Interagency Forum on Aging-Related Statistics. (2000). *Older Americans 2000: Key indicators of well-being.* Washington, DC: U.S. Government Printing Office.

Feimer, N. R. (1984). Environmental perception: The effects of media, evaluative context, and observer sample. *Journal of Environmental Psychology,* 4(1), 61–80.

Fisher, T. R. (2000). *In the scheme of things: Alternative thinking on the practice of architecture.* Minneapolis: University of Minnesota Press.

Fitzgerald, S. L. (2004, January/February). Back in the saddle: After a bumpy ride, assisted living begins to re-emerge as lenders' darling. *Assisted Living Today,* pp. 14–16.

Frank, J. (1999). "I live here, but it's not my home": Residents' experiences in assisted living. In B. Schwarz and R. Brent (Eds.), *Aging, autonomy and architecture: Advances in assisted living* (pp. 166–182). Baltimore: Johns Hopkins University Press.

Frank, J. B. (2002). *The paradox of aging in place in assisted living.* Westport, CT: Bergin & Garvey.

Frewald, D. B. (1989). *Preferences for older buildings: A psychological approach to architectural design.* Unpublished doctoral dissertation, University of Michigan.

Gans, H. (1974). *Popular culture and high culture: An analysis and evaluation of taste.* New York: Basic Books.

Gibson, M. J., Freiman, M., Gregory, S., Kassner, E., Kochera, A., Mullen, F., Pandya, S., Redfoot, D., Straight, A., and Wright, B. (2003). *Beyond 50.03: A report to the nation on independent living and disability.* Washington, DC: AARP.

Gitlin, L. N., Liebman, J., and Winter, L. (2003). Are environmental interventions effective in the management of Alzheimer's disease and related disorders? A synthesis of the evidence. *Alzheimer's Care Quarterly,* 4(2), 85–107.

Golant, S. M. (1998). Assisted living. In W. van Vliet (Ed.), *The encyclopedia of housing* (pp. 25–27). Thousand Oaks, CA: Sage Publications.

Golant, S. M. (1999). The promise of assisted living as a shelter and care alternative for frail American elders: A cautionary essay. In B. Schwarz and R. Brent (Eds.), *Aging, autonomy and architecture: Advances in assisted living* (pp. 32–59). Baltimore: Johns Hopkins University Press.

Greene, A., Hawes, C., Wood, M., and Woodsong, C. (1998). How do family members define quality in assisted living facilities? *Generations,* 21(4), 34–36.

Greenwood, D. J., and Levin, M. (1998). *Introduction to action research: Social research for social change.* Thousand Oaks, CA: Sage Publications.

Groat, L. (1982). Meaning in post-modern architecture: An examination using the multiple sorting task. *Journal of Environmental Psychology,* 2, 2–22.

Groat, L., and Wang, D. (2002). *Architectural research methods.* New York: John Wiley & Sons.

Harris, R., and Dyson, E. (2001). Recruitment of frail older people to research: Lessons learnt through experience. *Journal of Advanced Nursing,* 36(5), 643–651.

Hasell, M. J., and King, J. (in press). Social dimensions of the interiors of tall buildings. In A. D. Siedel and T. Heath (Eds.), *Social effects of the building environment.* London: Chapman Hall.

Hershberger, R. G. (1988). A study of meaning and architecture. In J. L. Nasar (Ed.), *Environmental aesthetics: Theory, research, and application* (pp. 175–194). New York: Cambridge University Press.

Hershberger, R. G., and Cass, R. (1988). Predicting user responses to buildings. In J. L. Nasar (Ed.), *Environmental aesthetics: Theory, research, and application* (pp. 195–227). New York: Cambridge University Press.

Herzog, T. R., and Gale, T. A. (1996). Preference for urban buildings as a function of age and nature context. *Environment and Behavior,* 28(1), 44–72.

Herzog, T. R., and Shier, R. L. (2000). Complexity, age, and building preference. *Environment and Behavior,* 32(4), 557–575.

Hetzel, L., and Smith, A. (2001). *The 65 years and over population: 2000.* Washington, DC: U.S. Census Bureau.

Hillier, B. (1996). *Space is the machine.* New York: Cambridge University Press.

Hoglund, D. J., and Ledewitz, S. D. (1999). Designing to meet the needs of people with Alzheimer's disease. In B. Schwarz and R. Brent (Eds.), *Aging, autonomy and architecture: Advances in assisted living* (pp. 229–261). Baltimore: Johns Hopkins University Press.

Hubbard, P. (1994). Professional vs lay tastes in design control—an empirical investigation. *Planning Practice and Research,* 9, 271–287.

Hyde, J. (2001). Understanding the context of assisted living. In K. H. Namazi and P. K. Chafetz (Eds.), *Assisted living: Current issues in facility management and resident care* (pp. 15–28). Westport, CT: Auburn House.

International Building Code (IBC). (2000). *International building code 2000.* Falls Church, VA: International Code Council.

Jacobson, J., Silverstein, M., and Winslow, B. (2002). *Patterns of home: The ten essentials of enduring design.* Newtown, CT: Taunton Press.

Kaplan, R. (1985). Nature at the doorstep: Residential satisfaction and the nearby environment. *Journal of Architectural and Planning Research,* 2, 115–127.

Kaplan, R. (1993). The role of nature in the context of the workplace. *Landscape and Urban Planning,* 26, 193–201.

Kaplan, R. (2001). The nature of the view from home: Psychological benefits. *Environment and Behavior,* 33(4), 507–542.

Kaplan, R., and Kaplan, S. (1995). *The experience of nature: A psychological perspective.* Ann Arbor: Ulrich's.

Kaplan, S., and Kaplan, R. (1978). *Humanscape: Environments for people.* Ann Arbor: Ulrich's. (Reprinted 1982).

Kaplan, S., and Kaplan, R. (1982). *Cognition and environment: Functioning in an uncertain world.* Ann Arbor: Ulrich's.

Kaplan, S., and Kaplan, R. (1989). The visual environment: Public participation in design and planning. *Journal of Social Issues,* 45(1), 59–86.

Kaplan, R., Kaplan, S., and Ryan, R. (1998). *With people in mind: Design and management of everyday nature.* Washington, DC: Island Press.

Kaplan, S., Kaplan, R., and Wendt, J. S. (1972). Rated preferences and complexity for natural and urban visual material. *Perception and Psychophysics,* 12, 354–356.

Kavanaugh, G. (1983). Foreword. In C. W. Moore, K. Smith, and P. Becker (Eds.), *Home sweet home* (pp. 11–13). New York: Rizzoli International Publications.

Kemp, J. (1987). *American vernacular: Regional influences in architecture and interior design.* New York: Viking Penguin.

Koss, E., and Gilmore, G. C. (1998). Environmental interventions and functional ability of AD patients. In B. Vellas, J. Filten, and G. Frisoni (Eds.), *Research and practice in Alzheimer's disease* (pp. 185–191). New York: Springer.

Lang, J. (1987). *Creating architectural theory: The role of the behavioral sciences in environmental design.* New York: Van Nostrand Reinhold.

Lang, J. (1988). Symbolic aesthetics in architecture: Toward a research agenda. In J. L. Nasar (Ed.), *Environmental Aesthetics: Theory, research, and application* (pp. 11–26). New York: Cambridge University Press.

Lavizzo-Mourey, R. J., Zinn, J., and Taylor, L. (1992). Ability of surrogates to represent satisfaction of nursing home residents with quality of care. *Journal of the American Geriatrics Society,* 40, 39–47.

Lawton, M. P. (1987). Methods in environmental research with older people. In R. B. Bechtel, R. W. Marans, and W. Michelson (Eds.), *Methods in environmental and behavioral research* (pp. 337–360). New York: Van Nostrand Reinhold.

Lawton, M. P. (2001). The physical environment of the person with Alzheimer's disease. *Aging and Mental Health,* 5(Suppl. 1), S56–S64.

Levin, C. E. (2001). *Resident and family perspectives on assisted living.* Unpublished doctoral dissertation, University of Minnesota.

Lynch, K. (1960). *The image of the city.* Cambridge: MIT Press.

Marsden, J. P. (1999). Older persons' and family members' perceptions of assisted living. *Environment and Behavior,* 31(1), 84–106.

Marsden, J. P. (2001). A framework for understanding homelike character in the context of assisted living housing. In B. Schwarz (Ed.), *Assisted living: Sobering realities* (pp. 79–96). New York: Haworth Press. Copublished simultaneously in *Journal of Housing for the Elderly,* 15(1/2), 2001.

Marsden, J. P., and Kaplan, R. (1999). Communicating homeyness from the outside: Elderly people's perceptions of assisted living. In B. Schwarz and R. Brent (Eds.), *Aging, autonomy and architecture: Advances in assisted living* (pp. 207–228). Baltimore: Johns Hopkins University Press.

Marsden, J. P., Briller, S. H., Calkins, M. P., and Proffitt, M. A. (2001). *Enhancing iden-*

tity and sense of home, Vol. 4 in M. P. Calkins, *Creating successful dementia care settings* (series). Baltimore: Health Professions Press.

Marsden, J. P., Meehan, R. A., and Calkins, M. P. (2001). Therapeutic kitchens for residents with dementia. *American Journal of Alzheimer's Disease and Other Dementias,* 16(5), pp. 303–311.

Marsden, J. P., Meehan, R. A., and Calkins, M. P. (2002). Activity-based kitchens for residents with dementia: Design strategies that support group activities. *Activities Directors' Quarterly for Alzheimer's and Other Dementias,* 3(3), pp. 15–22.

Martin, A. (2003, June). State of the industry. *Assisted Living Today,* pp. 20–24.

Materiality and resistance. (1994, May). *Architectural Review,* 194, pp. 4–5.

McCracken, G. (1989). Homeyness: A cultural account of the constellation of consumer goods and meanings. In E. Hirschman (Ed.), *Interpretive consumer culture* (pp. 168–183). Provo, UT: Association for Consumer Research.

McLean, B. (1996, December 23). Promising industries for 1997. *Fortune,* 134, 156–158.

MetLife Mature Market Institute. (2002). *MetLife survey of nursing home and home care costs 2002.* Westport, CT: Metropolitan Life Insurance.

Mitchell, J. M., and Kemp, B. J. (2000). Quality of life in assisted living homes: A multidimensional analysis. *Journal of Gerontology: Psychological Sciences,* 55B(2), 117–127.

Mollica, R. L. (2001). State policy and regulations. In S. Zimmerman, P. D. Sloane, and J. K. Eckert (Eds.), *Assisted living: Needs, practices, and policies in residential care for the elderly* (pp. 9–33). Baltimore: Johns Hopkins University Press.

Moore, C., and Allen, G. (1976). *Dimensions: Space, shape and scale in architecture.* New York: Architectural Record Books.

Moore, C., Allen, G., and Lyndon, D. (1974). *The place of houses.* New York: Holt, Rinehart & Winston.

Moore, J. (1998). *Assisted living 2000: Practical strategies for the next millennium.* Fort Worth: Westridge Press.

Moore, K. D. (1999). *Towards a language of assisted living: Understanding the physical setting through benchmarking.* Milwaukee: Center for Architecture & Urban Planning Research, University of Wisconsin–Milwaukee.

Mutran, E. J., Sudha, D., Reed, P. S., Menon, M., and Desai, T. (2001). African American use of residential care in North Carolina. In S. Zimmerman, P. D. Sloane, and J. K. Eckert (Eds.), *Assisted living: Needs, practices, and policies in residential care for the elderly* (pp. 92–114). Baltimore: Johns Hopkins University Press.

Namazi, K. H., and Chafetz, P. K. (2001). The concept, the terminology, and the occupants. In K. H. Namazi and P. K. Chafetz (Eds.), *Assisted living: Current issues in facility management and resident care* (pp. 1–11). Westport, CT: Auburn House.

Nasar, J. L. (1989). Symbolic meanings of house styles. *Environment and Behavior,* 21, 235–257.

Nasar, J. L. (1997). *The evaluative image of the city.* Beverly Hills, CA: Sage.

Nasar, J. L. (1999). *Design by competition: Making design competitions work.* New York: Cambridge University Press.

Nassauer, J. I. (1995). Messy ecosystem, orderly frames. *Landscape Journal,* 14(2), 161–170.

National Center for Assisted Living (NCAL). (2001). *Facts and trends: The assisted living sourcebook 2001.* Washington, DC: American Health Care Association and NCAL.

National Investment Conference (NIC). (1998). *National survey of assisted living residents: Who is the customer?* Annapolis, MD: NIC.

Nicol, D., and Pilling, S. (Eds.) (2000). *Changing architectural education: Towards a new professionalism.* New York: Spon Press.

Noell-Waggoner, E. (2002). Light: An essential intervention for Alzheimer's disease. *Alzheimer's Care Quarterly,* 3(4), 343–352.

Nowakowski, H. M. (2001, April). IAR Report. *ACSA News,* pp. 4, 7.

Orr, F. (1985). *Scale in architecture.* New York: Van Nostrand Reinhold.

Perez, K., Proffitt, M. A., and Calkins, M. P. (2001). *Minimizing disruptive behaviors,* Vol. 3 in M. P. Calkins, *Creating successful dementia care settings* (series). Baltimore: Health Professions Press.

Polyak, I. (2000). The center of attention. *American Demographics, 22*(11), 30–32.

Purcell, A. T. (1995). Experiencing American and Australian high- and popular-style houses. *Environment and Behavior, 27,* 771–800.

Purcell, A. T., and Nasar, J. L. (1992). Experiencing other people's houses: A model of similarities and differences in environmental experience. *Journal of Environmental Psychology, 12,* 199–211.

Rapoport, A. (1969). *House, form and culture.* Englewood Cliffs, NJ: Prentice-Hall.

Regnier, V. (1994). *Assisted living housing for the elderly: Design innovations from the United States and Europe.* New York: Van Nostrand Reinhold.

Regnier, V. (1999). The definition and evolution of assisted living within a changing system of long-term care. In B. Schwarz and R. Brent (Eds.), *Aging, autonomy and architecture: Advances in assisted living* (pp. 3–20). Baltimore: Johns Hopkins University Press.

Regnier, V. (2002). *Design for assisted living: Guidelines for housing the physically and mentally frail.* New York: John Wiley & Sons.

Regnier, V., Hamilton, J., and Yatabe, S. (1995). *Assisted living for the aged and frail: Innovations in design, management, and financing.* New York: Columbia University Press.

Rodriguez, B. (1994). Architects, nonarchitects and the image of the single-family house: Evaluations and preferences. In A. D. Seidel (Ed.), *Banking on design? Proceedings of the Twenty-fifth Annual Conference of the Environmental Design Research Association* (pp. 183–194). San Antonio, TX: Environmental Design Research Association.

Rylan, E. V. (1995). *Impact of interior design on the dining abilities of the elderly residents in assisted living and nursing homes.* Unpublished doctoral dissertation, Virginia Polytechnic Institute & State University.

Saint, A. (1983). *The image of the architect.* New Haven, CT: Yale University Press.

Sanoff, H. (2000). *Community participation methods in design and planning.* New York: John Wiley & Sons.

Schellhardt, T. D. (1997, February 18). This office building is a work of art. *Wall Street Journal,* p. A12.

Schwarz, B. (1999). Assisted living: An evolving place type. In B. Schwarz and R. Brent (Eds.), *Aging, autonomy and architecture: Advances in assisted living* (pp. 185–206). Baltimore: Johns Hopkins University Press.

Schwarz, B., and Brent, R. (1999a). *Aging, autonomy and architecture: Advances in assisted living.* Baltimore: Johns Hopkins University Press.

Schwarz, B., and Brent, R. (1999b). Emerging themes, further reflections. In B. Schwarz and R. Brent (Eds.), *Aging, autonomy and architecture: Advances in assisted living* (pp. 291–306). Baltimore: Johns Hopkins University Press.

Schwarz, B., Chaudhury, H., Brent, R., Cooney, T., Dunne, K., and Bostick, J. (2001). *Impact of design interventions in nursing home on residents with dementia, their families, and the staff.* Milwaukee: Center for Architecture & Urban Planning Research, University of Wisconsin–Milwaukee.

Sekulski, R., Jones, L., and Pastalan, L. A. (1999). A day's journey through life: An assessment game. In E. Steinfeld and G. S. Danford (Eds.), *Enabling environments: Measuring the impact of environment on disability and rehabilitation.* New York: Kluwer Academic/Plenum Publishers.

Sikorska, E. (1999). Organizational determinants of resident satisfaction with assisted living. *Gerontologist, 39*(4), 450–456.

Silverman, M., Ricci, E., Saxton, J., Ledewitz, S., McAllister, C., and Keane, C. (1996). *Woodside Place: The first three years of a residential Alzheimer's facility,* 2 vols. Oakmont, PA: Presbyterian SeniorCare.

Sloane, P. D., Zimmerman, S., and Walsh, J. F. (2001). The physical environment. In S. Zimmerman, P. D. Sloane, and J. K. Eckert (Eds.), *Assisted living: Needs, practices, and policies in residential care for the elderly* (pp. 173–197). Baltimore: Johns Hopkins University Press.

Smith, D. (2003). *The older population in the United States: March 2002.* Washington, DC: U.S. Census Bureau.

Snyder, J. (1984). *Architectural research.* New York: Van Nostrand Reinhold.

Sommer, R. (1983). *Social design: Creating buildings with people in mind.* Englewood Cliffs, NJ: Prentice-Hall.

Stamps, A. (1990). Use of photographs to stimulate environments: A meta-analysis. *Perceptual and Motor Skills,* 71, 907–913.

Stamps, A. (1991). Comparing preferences of neighbors and a neighborhood design review board. *Environment and Behavior,* 23, 618–629.

Stamps, A. (1997). Of time and preference: Temporal stability of environmental preferences. *Perceptual and Motor Skills,* 85, 883–896.

Talbot, J. F., and Kaplan, R. (1991). The benefits of nearby nature for elderly apartment residents. *International Journal of Aging and Human Development,* 33, 119–130.

Thomas, W. (1996). *Life worth living: How someone you love can still enjoy life in a nursing home.* Acton, MA: VanderWyk & Burnham.

Tinsley, R. K., and Warren, K. E. (1999). Assisted living: The current state of affairs. In B. Schwarz and R. Brent (Eds.), *Aging, autonomy and architecture: Advances in assisted living* (pp. 21–31). Baltimore: Johns Hopkins University Press.

Turnbull, A. (2001). *Empowerment and autonomy among continuing care nursing/ residents.* Unpublished master's thesis, University of Alberta.

Tzamir, Y., and Churchman, A. (1989). An ethical perspective on knowledge in architectural education. *Journal of Architectural and Planning Research,* 6(3), 227–239.

Ulrich, R. S. (1984). View through a window may influence recovery from surgery. *Science,* 224, 420–421.

Ulrich, R. S. (1995). Effects of healthcare interior design on wellness: Theory and recent scientific research. In S. Marberry (Ed.), *Innovations in healthcare design* (pp. 88–104). New York: Van Nostrand Reinhold.

Uman, G. C., Hocevar, D., Urman, H. N., Young, R., Hirsch, M., and Kohler, S. (2000). Satisfaction surveys with the cognitively impaired. In J. Cohen-Mansfield, F. K. Ejaz, and P. Werner (Eds.), *Satisfaction surveys in long-term care* (pp. 166–186). New York: Springer Publishing.

U.S. Administration on Aging. (2004). *Older population by age, 1900 to 2050.* www.aoa.gov/prof/statistics/online_stat_data/popage2050.xls; accessed August 23, 2004.

U.S. Department of Labor Bureau of Labor Statistics. (2003). *Demographic characteristics of the labor force.* www.bls.gov/cps/home.htm; accessed August 23, 2004.

Verderber, S. (1986). Dimensions of person-window transactions in the hospital environment. *Environment and Behavior,* 18, 450–466.

Verderber, S., and Refuerzo, B. (1999). On the construction of research-based design: A community health center. *Journal of Architectural and Planning Research,* 16(3), 225–241.

Verderber, S., and Refuerzo, B. J. (2003). Research-based architecture and the community healthcare consumer: A statewide initiative. *Journal of Architectural and Planning Research,* 20(1), 57–67.

Vischer, J. (2001). Post-occupancy evaluation: A multifaceted tool for building improvement. In Federal Facilities Council (Ed.), *Learning from our buildings: A state-of-the-practice summary of post-occupancy evaluation* (pp. 23–34). Washington, DC: National Academy Press.

Wang, D. (2003). Categories of ACSA conference papers: A critical evaluation of architectural research in light of social science methodological frameworks. *Journal of Architectural Education,* 56(4), 50–56.

Wilson, M. A. (1996). The socialization of architectural preference. *Journal of Environmental Psychology,* 16, 33–44.

Wolfe, T. (1981). *From Bauhaus to our house.* New York: Farrar, Straus, Giroux.

Wright, F. L. (1954). *The natural house.* New York: Horizon Press.

Zavotka, S. L., and Teaford, M. H. (1997). The design of shared social spaces in assisted living residences for older adults. *Journal of Interior Design,* 23(2), 2–16.

Zeisel, J. (1984). *Inquiry by design: Tools for environment-behavior research.* New York: Cambridge University Press.

Zeisel, J. (1999). *Housing options for people with dementia.* Canada Mortgage & Housing Corp.

Zeisel, J. (2003). Marketing therapeutic environments for Alzheimer's care. *Journal of Architectural and Planning Research,* 20(1), 75–86.

Zimmerman, S., Sloane, P. D., and Eckert, J. K. (2001a). *Assisted living: Needs, practices, and policies in residential care for the elderly.* Baltimore: Johns Hopkins University Press.

Zimmerman, S., Sloane, P. D., and Eckert, J. K. (2001b). Emerging issues in residential care/assisted living. In S. Zimmerman, P. D. Sloane, and J. K. Eckert (Eds.), *Assisted living: Needs, practices, and policies in residential care for the elderly* (pp. 317–331). Baltimore: Johns Hopkins University Press.

Zimring, C. (2002). Post occupancy evaluation: Issues and implementation. In R. B. Bechtel and A. Churchman (Eds.), *Handbook of environmental psychology* (pp. 306–319). New York: John Wiley & Sons.

INDEX

Page numbers followed by *f* indicate illustrations.

within, 40, 42, 55, 102; overhang of, 40; pitched, 39, 40, 52, 53, 53f, 55, 102; as shelter, 40, 55–56; tile, 60

rugs, 71. *See also* carpeting

safety, 11, 22, 38, 40, 54

SAGE. *See* Society for the Advancement of Gerontological Environments

scale, 41, 48–49. *See also* human scale

seating, 56–57, 67, 78, 78f, 79–80, 80f. *See also* chairs; couches/sofas

security, 38, 40, 54

sensory changes, 15, 43, 68, 69, 72, 90

services. *See* assisted living

shade, 57, 71

shades, window, 95, 104

shrubs, 40, 53, 54f, 57f, 58, 60, 62

sidewalks, 57

single-family house, 14, 39, 51–52, 63, 65–66, 73–74, 80, 85–86, 102

site, 42, 44, 53, 62

skylights, 90, 92, 93, 94–95, 95f, 98–99, 103, 104

social context, 24

social interaction, 38, 41, 103; in dining rooms, 85, 88, 92, 94f, 98; in living rooms, 79, 82; outdoors, 56–57

Society for the Advancement of Gerontological Environments (SAGE), 18

sofas/couches, 67, 74, 74f, 76f, 77f, 78, 83, 104. *See also* seating

sorting task, 3, 30–31

space: arrangement of, 39, 41, 42, 43; definition of, 66–67, 75–77, 103; use

of, 4, 22, 38, 43, 47, 63, 73; volume, 42, 69

staff, 4, 11, 34, 63, 90, 103

stimulation, 38, 39, 68, 72, 80

storage, 65

supportiveness of buildings, 1, 101

symbols, 39, 52

tablecloths, 85, 87f, 88, 91, 95, 97, 103

table finishes, 95, 96f

table lamps, 65f, 66, 74, 74f

tables: dining, 87f, 88, 89f, 94f, 97, 98, 102, 103; entry, 70, 72; game, 79, 80f, 103; picnic, 57

table settings, 85, 87f, 88–90, 91, 97, 103

television, 76f, 78, 79, 80f, 103

TESS-RC. *See* Therapeutic Environmental Screening Survey for Residential Care

theory: normative, 38; positive, 38

Therapeutic Environmental Screening Survey for Residential Care (TESS-RC), 22

therapeutic kitchens, 92

trees, 40, 43, 56f, 57f, 62, 62f

units, resident, 4, 52–53

urban design, 4

upholstery, 73, 85

usability, 102, 104; in conceptual framework, 42–43; in dining rooms, 86, 90, 92–98; for exteriors, 47, 50, 51, 57, 58, 59; in interior entries, 69, 70–71; in living rooms, 73–74, 80, 81–83

U.S. Bureau of the Census, 10

U.S. Senate Special Committee on Aging, 12

vegetation, 40, 43, 53, 56f, 62

views, 62; from circulation paths, 86–87, 89f; from doorways, 41, 65f, 71–72, 78, 78f; into a space, 75–76, 76f; between spaces, 65f, 66, 67, 68f, 102; from window, 41, 43–44, 53, 54, 61, 77, 79, 83, 95, 98–99, 104

visual access. *See* views

wall coverings / finishes, 43, 66, 73, 85

walls, 40, 74, 76f, 95, 95f, 102

water, 43

well-being, 33–34

window boxes, 41

windows: bay, 41, 54, 55f, 56f; bow, 54; clerestory, 92, 93, 94–95, 94f, 103, 104; height from ground, 61; open, 41, 57, 102; panes, 40, 61, 74f, 81; shades for, 95, 104; shapes and sizes, 39, 52, 53f, 60, 61, 102, 103

window seats, 41

window shutters, 41, 52, 53, 53f, 58, 59f, 102

window treatments, 73, 74, 74f, 85, 86, 87f, 102; curtains, 41, 57, 65f, 66, 87f, 89f, 95, 104; shades, 95, 104

Woodside Place, 22

Wright, Frank Lloyd, 29, 40, 42, 68

zoning, 14–15